The Dysvascular and Diabetic Patient: Update in Diagnosis, Treatment and Rehabilitation

Guest Editor

KEVIN N. HAKIMI, MD

PHYSICAL MEDICINE AND REHABILITATION CLINICS OF NORTH AMERICA

www.pmr.theclinics.com

Consulting Editor
GEORGE H. KRAFT, MD, MS

November 2009 • Volume 20 • Number 4

SAUNDERS an imprint of ELSEVIER, Inc.

W.B. SAUNDERS COMPANY
A Division of Elsevier Inc.

1600 John F. Kennedy Boulevard • Suite 1800 • Philadelphia, Pennsylvania 19103

http://www.theclinics.com

PHYSICAL MEDICINE AND REHABILITATION CLINICS OF NORTH AMERICA Volume 20, Number 4
November 2009 ISSN 1047-9651, ISBN-10: 1-4377-1263-0, ISBN-13: 978-1-4377-1263-6

Editor: Debora Dellapena
Developmental Editor: Theresa Collier

Reprints. For copies of 100 or more of articles in this publication, please contact the Commercial Reprints Department, Elsevier Inc., 360 Park Avenue South, New York, NY 10010-1710. Tel.: 212-633-3812; Fax: 212-462-1935; E-mail: reprints@elsevier.com.

Physical Medicine and Rehabilitation Clinics of North America (ISSN 1047-9651) is published quarterly by Elsevier Inc., 360 Park Avenue South, New York, NY 10010-1710. Months of publication are February, May, August, and November. Periodicals postage paid at New York, NY and additional mailing offices. Subscription price per year is $213.00 (US individuals), $339.00 (US institutions), $107.00 (US students), $259.00 (Canadian individuals), $443.00 (Canadian institutions), $155.00 (Canadian students), $319.00 (foreign individuals), $443.00 (foreign institutions), and $155.00 (foreign students). Foreign air speed delivery is included in all *Clinics* subscription prices. All prices are subject to change without notice. **POSTMASTER:** Send address changes to *Physical Medicine and Rehabilitation Clinics of North America*, Elsevier Health Sciences Division, Subscription Customer Service, 3251 Riverport Lane, Maryland Heights, MO 63043. **Customer Service: Telephone: 1-800-654-2452 (U.S. and Canada); 314-447-8871 (outside U.S. and Canada). Fax: 314-447-8029. E-mail: journalscustomerservice-usa@elsevier.com (for print support); journalsonlinesupport-usa@elsevier.com (for online support).**

Physical Medicine and Rehabilitation Clinics of North America is indexed in *Excerpta Medica, MEDLINE/ PubMed (Index Medicus), Cinahl, and Cumulative Index to Nursing and Allied Health Literature.*

Printed and bound in the United Kingdom
Transferred to Digital Print 2011

Contributors

CONSULTING EDITOR

GEORGE H. KRAFT, MD, MS
Alvord Professor of Multiple Sclerosis Research; Professor, Rehabilitation Medicine;
Adjunct Professor, Neurology, University of Washington School of Medicine, Seattle,
Washington

GUEST EDITOR

KEVIN N. HAKIMI, MD
Assistant Professor, Department of Rehabilitation Medicine, University of Washington
School of Medicine; Outpatient Director, Rehabilitation Care Services, Veterans Affairs
Puget Sound Health Care System, Seattle, Washington

AUTHORS

JENNIFER DOROSZ, MD
Assistant Professor of Medicine, Division of Cardiology, University of Colorado, Cardiac
& Vascular Center, Anschutz Inpatient Pavilion, Aurora, Colorado

KEVIN N. HAKIMI, MD
Assistant Professor, Department of Rehabilitation Medicine, University of Washington
School of Medicine; Outpatient Director, Rehabilitation Care Services, Veterans Affairs
Puget Sound Health Care System, Seattle, Washington

MICHAEL HENRY, MD
Attending Physician, Department of Medicine, Division of Infectious Diseases,
Bronx-Lebanon Hospital Center, Bronx, New York

ILEANA M. HOWARD, MD
Clinical Assistant Professor, Department of Rehabilitation Medicine, University
of Washington, Seattle, Washington

MARK P. JENSEN, PhD
Department of Rehabilitation Medicine, University of Washington School of Medicine;
Multidisciplinary Pain Center, University of Washington Medical Center,
Seattle, Washington

ANDY O. MILLER, MD
Attending Physician, Department of Medicine, Division of Infectious Diseases,
Bronx-Lebanon Hospital Center, Bronx, New York

TRAVIS L. OSBORNE, PhD
Department of Rehabilitation Medicine, University of Washington School of Medicine;
Anxiety and Stress Reduction Center of Seattle, Seattle, Washington

KATHERINE A. RAICHLE, PhD
Department of Rehabilitation Medicine, University of Washington School of Medicine; Department of Psychology, Seattle University, Seattle, Washington

ELIZABETH V. RATCHFORD, MD
Director, Johns Hopkins Center for Vascular Medicine; Assistant Professor of Medicine, Department of Medicine, Division of Cardiology, Johns Hopkins University School of Medicine, Baltimore, Maryland

MAYA J. SALAMEH, MD
Director, Cardiovascular Ultrasound Laboratory, Columbia University Medical Center; Assistant Professor of Clinical Medicine, Department of Medicine, Division of Cardiology, Columbia University College of Physicians and Surgeons, New York, New York

JELENA N. SVIRCEV, MD
Staff Physician, Department of Veterans Affairs, Spinal Cord Injury Service, Puget Sound Health Care System; Clinical Assistant Professor, Department of Rehabilitation Medicine, University of Washington, Seattle, Washington

HEIKKI UUSTAL, MD
Chief of Rehabilitation Services, St. Peter's University Hospital, New Brunswick, New Jersey

KAREN WOOTEN, MD
Clinical Assistant Professor, Department of Rehabilitation Medicine, University of Washington; Attending Physician, Rehabilitative Care Services, Veterans Affairs Puget Sound Health Care System, Seattle, Washington

Contents

Diabetic foot ulcerations are a costly and common public health challenge. Although several organizations have emphasized the need to increase awareness of this problem and called health care providers to action to decrease the incidence of ulceration and amputation, there is limited evidence regarding what interventions are best suited to accomplish this goal. This article reviews the pathogenesis, risk factors, and current interventions that have been studied for the prevention of foot ulceration. Preventive measures with evidence for decreasing incidence of ulceration include patient education, offloading abnormal pressures with foot orthotics, and thermal monitoring.

Foot infections are a major cause of morbidity and mortality in diabetics. Evaluation of diabetic foot infections often requires clinical, radiologic, laboratory, and microbiologic assessment. Osteomyelitis has a profound impact on the prognosis and management of these infections, and diagnosis can be difficult; the gold standard remains bone biopsy. Despite a panoply of studies, the optimal management of diabetic foot infections remains poorly understood. Antibiotics, surgery, rehabilitation and/or off-loading, and glycemic control remain the cornerstones of treatment; alternative therapies remain largely unproven.

The prevalence of peripheral arterial disease is high and will continue to grow with our aging population. It is often under diagnosed and under treated due to a general lack of awareness on the part of the patient and the practitioner. The evidence-base is growing for the optimal medical management of the patient with peripheral arterial disease; in parallel, endovascular revascularization options continue to improve. Exercise training for claudication rehabilitation plays a critical role. Comprehensive care of the peripheral arterial disease patient focuses on the ultimate goals of improving quality of life and reducing cardiovascular morbidity and mortality.

Diabetic peripheral neuropathy (DPN) is a common disorder that can lead to limb loss and death. Up to 50% of DPN patients can be asymptomatic. This fact contributes to making DPN the leading cause of lower limb amputation. The degree of heterogeneity in the clinical manifestations of DPN makes diagnosing this condition difficult. This article reviews the characteristics, diagnosis, electrodiagnosis, classification, pathogenesis, and treatment of DPN.

Lower-extremity amputation secondary to dysvascular disease, including diabetes and peripheral vascular disease, is a major health problem in the United States. Due to the increased comorbidities in this patient population, pre-operative rehabilitation evaluation by a multidisciplinary team is crucial to ensure optimal patient outcomes. This article discusses the key factors that may affect functional outcomes in this patient population and outlines important history and physical examination components that should be evaluated pre-operatively.

Evaluation and management of diabetic and dysvascular patients with lower limb amputation begins with a thorough history and physical examination. A pre-prosthetic and prosthetic program of physical therapy, pain management, psychological assessment, and education helps patients resume functional mobility and gain acceptance of the limb loss. Physicians and prosthetic teams work together to design and prescribe the most appropriate prosthetic device for patients to reach maximal functional level. Careful monitoring of patients and a full understanding of patients' medical conditions help avoid complications and falls during rehabilitation. Long-term follow-up is necessary to assess fit and function of prosthetic devices.

Dysvascular and diabetic patients are faced with high rates of chronic pain as a consequence of numerous secondary sequelae, including diabetic neuropathy and limb loss. Researchers and scientists have put forth a tremendous amount of effort to understand the complex nature of pain in this population of individuals, as well as others with chronic pain secondary to illness and injury. The emergent understanding of anatomy and sensory physiology within the past century has fueled an initial focus of understanding pain from a purely neurologic and biochemical perspective. Over the past few decades, the field has moved toward an understanding of pain as a process involving the dynamic interaction of biologic, psychological, behavioral, and social variables. This article provides a brief

overview of several psychosocial processes, cognitive, affective, and behavioral, that have emerged as influential to the experience, impact, and
treatment of pain.

THE CLINICS ARE NOW AVAILABLE ONLINE!

Access your subscription at:
www.theclinics.com

Foreword

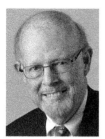

George H. Kraft, MD, MS
Consulting Editor

When I was in training, we received considerable experience in managing amputations. Typically, most lower limb amputations in the civilian population were due to peripheral vascular disease, and most from the military were traumatic. This was during the Vietnam War, and land mines were a source of nonrepairable injury to the lower limbs.

Fortunately, today land mine injuries are much more rare. And, with better management of diabetes and peripheral vascular disease, there are also fewer dysvascular lower limb amputations. Medical trainees and physicians newly entering practice have reduced opportunities to learn management skills for the dysvascular and diabetic patient.

So it is with appreciation that the *Physical Medicine and Rehabilitation Clinics of North America* can present this issue, guest-edited by Dr. Kevin Hakimi, on this topic. Both peripheral vascular disease from arteriosclerosis and small artery disease from diabetes can result in the same outcome: the dysvascular limb. These 2 causes lend themselves to many of the same management techniques and are included in this issue.

The best amputee management is, of course, to prevent amputation. No matter how sophisticated prosthetics become, they can never replace the original limb. The first step in this management cascade is the identification and management of skin breakdown and development of ulceration. If this fails, the ulcer must then be managed, and infection treated.

If limb salvage attempts fail, then amputation becomes a necessary consideration, and a preamputation assessment plan is necessary for optimal outcome of surgery. Then there is the prosthesis: above knee, below knee, or partial foot. This must be well chosen and matched to the needs and capacities of the patient.

Invariably, amputation takes both a physical and psychological toll. Both of these issues must be managed. Systemic vascular (eg, cardiac disease) and causative neurologic (eg, paraplegia) conditions must also be addressed. Finally, postamputation rehabilitation—physical and vocational—must be facilitated.

Phys Med Rehabil Clin N Am 20 (2009) ix–x
doi:10.1016/j.pmr.2009.07.001
1047-9651/09/$ – see front matter © 2009 Elsevier Inc. All rights reserved.

pmr.theclinics.com

It may not "take a village" to achieve all of this, but it certainly takes an integrated team. My thanks go to Dr. Hakimi for taking on this important but challenging issue.

George H. Kraft, MD, MS
Alvord Professor of MS Research
Professor, Rehabilitation Medicine
Adjunct Professor, Neurology
University of Washington
Box 356490, 1959 NE Pacific Street
Seattle, WA 98195-6490, USA

E-mail address:
ghkraft@uw.edu (G.H. Kraft)

Preface

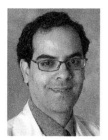

Kevin N. Hakimi, MD
Guest Editor

The number of patients with cardiovascular diseases, such as coronary heart disease and peripheral vascular diseases, and related conditions such as diabetes mellitus continues to increase in the United States. All these patients have diseases that cause ischemia and macro- and/or microvascular abnormalities, and thus they can all be grouped under the category of dysvascular diseases. All rehabilitation providers will encounter these patients in their practices regardless of their rehabilitation specialty, and they must have the tools to ensure that, after appropriate diagnosis, function is maximized through appropriate treatment and rehabilitation.

The relationship between diabetes, peripheral neuropathy, and lower-extremity amputation is well known. The rehabilitation provider may encounter these dysvascular patients initially during electrodiagnostic evaluations for peripheral neuropathy. The rehabilitation specialist should play a role in prevention of amputation as well as preoperative, postoperative, and prosthetic management. Patients with coronary heart disease and claudication secondary to peripheral vascular disease can benefit from structured exercise programs that are historically underused in the United States. Additionally, specific rehabilitation populations, such as those with spinal cord injury, may have unique presentations and require different treatment approaches.

This issue of *Physical Medicine and Rehabilitation Clinics of North America* is devoted to the patient with dysvascular disease. It covers several broad but interwoven topics, including diabetic foot ulcers, amputation, electrodiagnostics, peripheral vascular disease, cardiac rehabilitation, and pain.

I would like to acknowledge Dr Kraft for his mentorship during my residency and as a junior faculty member. I would also like to thank Dr Czerniecki, an expert in amputee care, who helped me formulate many of the concepts related to the dysvascular

doi:10.1016/j.pmr.2009.06.008
pmr.theclinics.com

patient. Lastly, I would like to acknowledge all the writers who contributed to this important issue.

Kevin N. Hakimi, MD
Assistant Professor
Department of Rehabilitation Medicine
University of Washington
Veterans Administration Puget Sound Health Care System
RCS-117, 1660 South Columbian Way
Seattle, WA 98108, USA

E-mail address:
khakimi@u.washington.edu (K.N. Hakimi)

The Prevention of Foot Ulceration in Diabetic Patients

Ileana M. Howard, MD

KEYWORDS

• Diabetic foot • Ulceration • Prevention • Patient education
• Orthotic devices

The prevalence of diabetes in the United States and worldwide is growing steadily, and with it the impact of diabetes-related morbidity is likewise growing and presenting new challenges for public health systems. In 2007, there were an estimated 23.6 million people in the United States living with diabetes mellitus, representing a 13.5% increase since 2005.[1] This trend is not limited to the United States alone, because the prevalence of type 2 diabetes mellitus and the economic stress of its associated complications is growing at a rapid rate globally. The growing burden of chronic disease is changing the face of health care and most profoundly affecting developing nations, where it is estimated that 80% of the world's 250 million persons with diabetes reside.[2,3]

Diabetic foot ulcerations and amputations are dreaded complications related to diabetes and have a severe impact on the individual and society. On an individual level, foot ulcers often represent a chronic disorder that may severely limit function, work capacity, and quality of life. On a public health scale, foot disorders represent a costly burden on the medical system as one of the leading causes for hospitalization in persons with diabetes. The rate of amputation in individuals with diabetes is 10 times higher than in persons without diabetes. Diabetes is associated with 60% of nontraumatic lower-limb amputations; in the United States, this represented 71 000 amputations in 2004.[1] Even if an ulcer heals with medical therapy, the recurrence rate in patients with diabetes remains high at nearly 70% within 5 years.[4]

Reducing the incidence of diabetic ulcerations and amputations has been pronounced a main public health goal for many years in the United States and abroad; however, despite the acknowledgment of this serious public health challenge, the number of amputations in persons with diabetes continues to rise, increasing 30% from 1980 to 1990.[5] One of the main challenges in reducing the incidence of diabetic foot ulcerations is in determining what interventions are most

Department of Rehabilitation Medicine, 1959 NE Pacific Street, Box 356490, University of Washington, Seattle, WA 98195, USA
E-mail address: ileana.howard@va.gov

Phys Med Rehabil Clin N Am 20 (2009) 595–609
doi:10.1016/j.pmr.2009.06.010
1047-9651/09/$ – see front matter. Published by Elsevier Inc.

pmr.theclinics.com

effective toward this end. Unfortunately, research in prevention is still somewhat sparse in comparison to the body of evidence for treatment. Many of the current practice guidelines are based on consensus and tradition rather than research and evidence-based medicine. The aim of this article is to outline the current understanding of the pathologic process underlying diabetic foot ulceration, the risk factors associated with the development of ulcers, and interventions that are in use or have been studied to modify this risk.

PATHOGENESIS OF DIABETIC FOOT ULCERS

The feet of patients with diabetes are at increased risk for ulceration because of the damaging effects of diabetic peripheral neuropathy. Ulceration is usually the end result of interplay between several component factors, including poor sensation, structural foot abnormalities, and local trauma. The course leading from hyperglycemia to neuropathy is not entirely understood, although neural hypoxia secondary to metabolic abnormalities of hyperglycemia and dyslipidemia may be a contributing factor.[6] Diabetic peripheral neuropathy is a length-dependent, mixed sensorimotor, demyelinating, and axonal process affecting multiple nerve fiber subtypes. The most well-known and common of these is sensory neuropathy, which leads to loss of protective sensation. Motor neuropathy also may produce intrinsic foot muscle atrophy and subsequent anatomic foot deformity, such as clawfoot, hammertoes, or Charcot foot. Range-of-motion limitations are also thought to result from direct glycosylation of tendons in the lower extremity.

The result of these foot deformities is abnormal weight-bearing distribution in the foot, which places high-pressure areas at risk for skin breakdown (**Fig. 1**). Finally, autonomic neuropathy decreases normal temperature and secretion regulation, which impairs the effectiveness of the skin barrier. Despite the extensive repercussions of diabetic neuropathy, ulcerations generally do not occur spontaneously in the foot of a patient with diabetes but occur as a result of local trauma in a predisposed foot. This may occur from local trauma caused by poor footwear or other external insult, such as trauma from nail clipping, falls, or repetitive trauma.

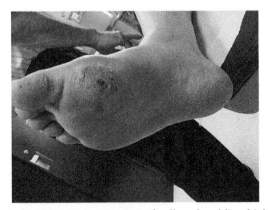

Fig. 1. Diabetic foot ulceration. Note presence of callous heralding high-pressure–bearing regions, particularly beneath the great toe, metatarsals, and calcaneous. (*Courtesy of Gregory Raugi, MD, Seattle, Washington.*)

Once an ulcer is present, healing may be impaired by the same factors that contributed to the initial ulceration, including elevated blood glucose and abnormal pressure distribution. Poor circulation and infection may further impede healing in patients with foot ulcerations. Multiple classification systems exist to describe diabetic ulcerations, the most common of which include the Warner classification system and the University of Texas system, which reports the depth and width and presence or absence of ischemia and infection.[7]

RISK FACTORS FOR FOOT ULCERATION IN PATIENTS WITH DIABETES

To design interventions for the prevention of diabetic foot ulceration and estimate a patient's risk of ulceration, multiple epidemiologic studies have evaluated cohorts of patients with diabetes to quantify the individual contributions of suspected clinical risk factors to lower extremity ulceration and amputation. The most consistently cited risk factors supported by evidence from prospective cross-sectional and case-control studies mirror the key elements in the pathogenesis of foot ulceration. This is witnessed by the systematic review and meta-analysis by Crawford and colleagues[8] in 2007, which cited clinical indicators of diabetic neuropathy (high vibratory perception threshold, impaired sensation to monofilament testing, absent ankle jerk reflexes, high plantar pressures), foot deformities (limited subtalar joint and first metatarsal-phalangeal joint range of motion), or established vascular disease (by history of prior ulceration or amputation) as significant predictors of ulceration (**Table 1**). Other proposed risk factors that predict ulceration with less consistent support from population studies include ankle-brachial index, HbA_{1C}, visual acuity, and duration of diabetes mellitus.[10]

Identified risk factors for amputation also include indicators of peripheral neuropathy (insensitivity to monofilament testing) and peripheral vascular disease (by history of prior lower extremity ulcers or lower extremity amputation). Other risk factors include peripheral vascular disease, which is measured by decreased transcutaneous oxygen pressure measurement ($TcPO_2 < 50$ mm Hg), and smoking, duration of diabetes, and treatment with insulin (**Table 2**).

Table 1			
Epidemiologic studies evaluating risk of ulceration			
Study, Publication Year	N	Design	Risk Factors Identified
Boyko, 2006	1285	Observational cohort study, mean follow-up 3.38 years	A_{1C} Impaired vision Prior foot ulcer Prior amputation Monofilament insensitivity Tinea pedis Onychomycosis
Frykberg, 1998[9]	251	Cross-sectional	High foot pressures > 6 kg/cm^2, Neuropathy by high VPT or insensitivity to imonofilament
Cowley, 2008	2939	Prospective	Hammer/claw toes Bony prominences Charcot/drop foot Hammer/claw toes Charcot/drop foot

Table 2
Epidemiologic studies evaluating risk of amputation

Study	N	Design	Risk Factors Identified
Reiber, 1992[11]	236	Case-control	ABI < 0.45 Decreased vibratory perception Low HDL No outpatient diabetes education
Adler, 1999[12]	776	Observational cohort study, mean follow-up 3.3 years	PVD defined as transcutaneous oxygen < 50 mm Hg Insensitivity to monofilament testing Lower extremity ulcers Prior lower extremity amputation Treatment with insulin when controlling for duration of diabetes and other factors in the model Foot ulcer PVD with decreased pulses or ABI ≤ 0.8
Samaan, 2008[13]	4778	Cross-sectional study	Age Years of disease duration Height Cigarette smoking

Abbreviation: ABI, ankle-brachial index.

INTERVENTIONS FOR THE PREVENTION OF DIABETIC FOOT ULCERATIONS
Glycemic Control

Given the connection among hyperglycemia, peripheral neuropathy, and ulceration, it calls to question whether improving blood glucose control may decrease the risk of ulcer formation. Epidemiologic studies have revealed correlation between glycemic control (measured as HbA_{1C} values) and the risk of developing foot ulcers[10] and lower extremity amputations.[12] A prospective, observational study by Stratton and colleagues[14] in 2000 revealed a linear association between HbA_{1C} values and incidence of amputation or death from peripheral vascular disease. Evidence indicates that aggressive glycemic control reduces the risk of developing peripheral neuropathy.[15] Unfortunately, no studies have specifically evaluated interventions designed to gauge the effect of improved glycemic control on incidence of ulceration; however, this intervention has been included in combined/complex interventions, which is discussed later in this article.

Evaluation and Treatment of Peripheral Arterial Disease

A common comorbidity that contributes to the risk of amputation in patients with diabetes is peripheral arterial disease (PAD). Risk factors for PAD include smoking, hypertension, hyperlipidemia, and longstanding diabetes. Although arterial insufficiency is rarely the sole cause of ulcer formation, it often delays or prevents ulcer healing in patients with diabetes. The diagnosis of PAD is based on clinical, physiologic, or radiographic evaluation. Clinic-based evaluation for PAD begins with palpation of peripheral pulses. Unfortunately, wide variation in clinical techniques leads to a low rate of interexaminer reliability. Peripheral pulses also may be impalpable in a small proportion of patients without vascular compromise. An ankle-brachial index is another appropriate and more reproducible screening tool to detect PAD; values of less than 0.9 suggest arterial insufficiency in the lower extremities. Unfortunately, atherosclerosis may cause a false elevation of the ankle-brachial index. Another quantitative tool for assessing peripheral circulation is transcutaneous oxygen pressure measurement ($TcPO_2$); a value of more than 40 to 50 mm Hg is considered normal.[16] Radiographically, peripheral arterial supply may be further assessed with angiography, MR angiography, CT angiography, or ultrasound.

Treatment for PAD is well described in the literature and may include smoking cessation, medications, or revascularization surgery. Although the treatment of PAD seems to aid wound healing in dysvascular patients, the role of this intervention in prevention of ulceration is unclear. No studies have evaluated the effect of revascularization alone on the incidence of ulceration.

Evaluation and Treatment of Peripheral Neuropathy

Diabetic neuropathy is one of the leading causes of foot ulceration, and it is estimated that 80% of patients with diabetes who have foot lesions have known peripheral neuropathy.[17] Numerous clinical tools are used to evaluate patients for peripheral neuropathy. Currently, the gold standard for clinic-based evaluation of sensory neuropathy in patients with diabetes is examination with a 10-g Semmes-Weinstein monofilament. Other useful clinical evaluation techniques include biothesiometry to determine vibratory perception threshold, ankle reflex testing, and clinical history and using a subjective neuropathy scoring system, such as the University of Texas Subjective Peripheral Neuropathy verbal questionnaire. All of these screening techniques seem to be sensitive for the determination of neuropathy and prediction of ulceration risk; the use of multiple screening techniques seems to increase specificity.[18] Electrodiagnosis can further confirm this condition and evaluate for peripheral nerve entrapment, such as tarsal tunnel syndrome, as a mimicking or coexisting condition.

Several medical therapies are under evaluation for treatment of diabetic neuropathy, although their impact on diabetic complications such as diabetic foot ulcers is unclear. Aggressive glycemic control has been associated with significant decreases in the incidence of peripheral neuropathy but has not been found to reverse the effects of neuropathy.[15] Various other pharmacologic interventions, such as the use of cilostazol, have been studied as possible means of treating diabetic neuropathy; however, the research in this area is still in preclinical stages.[19] Another class of medication currently being evaluated for effect on diabetic neuropathy is the statins.[20,21] In a study of rouvastatin on a diabetic rat model, use of this medication was associated with improvements in nerve conduction velocities.[6] These interventions are currently in preclinical stages for treatment of diabetic neuropathy, and the impact on diabetic complications also remains to be seen.

Peripheral nerve decompressive surgery has been proposed as a measure to improve protective sensation and decrease the risk of foot ulcer formation. The theory underlying this intervention is that persons with diabetes are more prone to peripheral nerve entrapment than patients without diabetes; peripheral nerve decompression may restore protective sensation and reduce the risk of ulceration. Commonly targeted nerves for surgical decompression in the lower extremities include the tibial nerve at the ankle, calcaneal, medial plantar, and lateral plantar nerves (tarsal tunnel release), and peroneal nerve at the ankle and knee. Unfortunately, there is no conclusive evidence that peripheral nerve decompression provides any significant benefit for peripheral neuropathy, as concluded in a recent systematic review by Chaudhry and colleagues.[22] This study reviewed 6 observational studies detailing treatment in a total of 218 patients; however, the included studies were heterogeneous in the preoperative objective diagnosis of peripheral neuropathy and the postoperative improvement measurement tools. A retrospective study by Aszmann and colleagues[23] followed 50 patients for a mean 4.5 years after peripheral nerve decompression surgery and reported decreased incidence of ulceration and amputation in the treated limb versus nontreated limb, with no ulcers or amputations in the treated limb, but 12 ulcers and 3 amputations in nontreated contralateral limbs.

Screening Foot Examination

The current standard of care for patients with diabetes includes an annual foot examination, during which the practitioner may evaluate for peripheral neuropathy, callus formation, onchomycosis, structural foot deformities, circulatory disturbances, wounds, and appropriateness of footwear.[24] Specific foot deformities that have been found to be predictive of lower extremity ulceration include hammer/claw foot deformities and structural deformities, such as Charcot foot and drop foot.[25] Regular foot examinations alone have not been found to decrease the incidence of lower extremity ulceration or amputation, however.[26] Regular foot examination may help identify patients at risk for ulceration, which allows the practitioner to stratify patients according to risk of ulceration to guide interventions and may reveal modifiable risk factors that can decrease the likelihood of ulceration. Patients often fail to identify early-stage wounds, causing delay in appropriate treatment. This is supported by a recent prospective, observational study, which determined that a significant percentage (39.7%) of foot ulcers was first identified by a health care professional rather than the patient or caregiver/relative.[27] The optimal frequency of screening foot examinations has not been established.

Evaluation and Treatment of Abnormal Plantar Pressure Distribution

Given that abnormal plantar pressure distribution is a known contributing factor to ulceration, monitoring and quantification of plantar pressures have been investigated as means of identifying patients at risk of ulceration and monitoring the effects of pressure-reducing interventions.[9,28] Plantar pressure monitoring takes many forms, from qualitative podoscopy to digital plantar pressure monitoring.[29] Pressure measurements may be performed on a static platform or mat or be measured with in-shoe inserts. Specific plantar pressure variables that have been used for predicting risk of ulceration include peak plantar pressure, pressure beneath the metatarsal heads, and forefoot-to-rearfoot plantar pressure ratio. In all cases, higher pressures are predictive of ulceration. In a prospective study by Caselli and colleagues,[28] an elevated forefoot-to-rearfoot ratio was seen only in severe peripheral neuropathy (as measured by the neuropathy disability score) and was associated with an increased likelihood of ulceration (OR 1.37; 1.16–1.61, $P < .0001$).

Once a patient has been found to be at increased risk of ulceration because of abnormal plantar pressure distribution, plantar pressure monitoring can be used to assess the efficacy of measures designed to redistribute plantar pressures. This is most commonly performed with specialized footwear, such as custom insoles (discussed later). Surgical correction has been evaluated for this purpose. For example, Achilles tendon lengthening has been proposed as an intervention to decrease forefoot pressures in patients with diabetic neuropathy and possibly diminish the risk of forefoot ulceration.[30]

Specialized Footwear

Custom footwear, including in-shoe orthotics and custom shoes, is the most common intervention for correction of abnormal pressure distribution in the feet of patients with diabetes and is a common clinical intervention used in an attempt to decrease the risk of ulcer formation. Despite the common usage of this intervention, however, the breadth of evidence relating therapeutic footwear for prevention rather than treatment of diabetic foot ulcers is surprisingly sparse.

The literature regarding primary ulcer prevention is limited, although several small studies do suggest that specialized footwear does confer benefit. A small, randomized trial by Colagiuri and colleagues[31] in 1995 found that custom-made foot orthotics improved the rates of resolution of callus, an indicator of abnormal pressure distribution in the foot. Although the primary outcome of this study was callus resolution and not ulcer prevention, this does demonstrate modification of risk factors in normalizing plantar pressure distribution. A systematic review by Bus and colleagues[32] in 2008 found no experimental studies on the role of footwear and offloading in primary ulcer prevention and mixed findings regarding the role of therapeutic shoes in secondary ulcer prevention. Another systematic review by Spencer in 2000 revealed callus resolution with offloading interventions but no studies demonstrating evidence of benefit of custom foot orthotics specifically for primary prevention of ulceration.[33]

Custom footwear does seem to decrease the risk of re-ulceration. A randomized, controlled trial by Uccioli and colleagues[34,35] in 1995 revealed that manufactured shoes significantly reduced the risk of re-ulceration in comparison to standard footwear. Another study by Busch and colleagues in 2003 reported similar benefits of specialized footwear in decreasing the incidence of re-ulceration. Although the evidence behind custom footwear for prevention of diabetic ulceration is limited, it remains a common intervention for patients deemed to be at higher risk of ulceration because of peripheral neuropathy or foot deformity. Specialized footwear is a covered benefit for patients with diabetes who have a history of amputation or peripheral neuropathy with callus or peripheral vascular disease under the Medicare Therapeutic Shoe Bill of 2004.

Patient Education

Diabetic foot education programs generally include instruction on daily foot self-inspection, avoidance of trauma, such as walking barefoot, and encouragement for patients to contact their physician should any new abnormality appear. Interventions aimed at educating patients on foot care and self-monitoring have been studied, with mixed results.[36] A systematic review published in 2001 by Valk and colleagues[37] revealed some evidence that a patient education program improves patient foot care and reported evidence supporting the effect of an patient education program on decreasing ulcer incidence and callous formation, particularly for high-risk patients (those with prior infection ulcer, or amputation) receiving intensive educational interventions. Other randomized, controlled trials included in this systematic review did not reveal similar effect of education on decreasing ulceration incidence.

A recent randomized control trial by Lincoln and colleagues[36] that evaluated individual educational sessions for patients with history of prior ulceration found improved compliance with recommended foot care behaviors but no significant difference in the incidence of recurrent ulceration in 12 months of follow-up between intervention and control groups. Patient education is often included in complex/combined intervention strategies. This makes it difficult to ascertain what proportion of the reported benefits can be ascribed to the educational component of these interventions, however.

Provider Education

In addition to educating patients on foot care and self-examination, several studies have highlighted the importance of provider education. The American Diabetes Association guidelines recommend that providers—at minimum—learn competency in performing a basic screening examination of the foot, including the associated neurologic, vascular, dermatologic, and musculoskeletal systems.[38] Despite adequate provider knowledge, another barrier to identifying patients at risk for ulceration lies in compliance with routine foot examinations. Prior observational studies note poor provider compliance with routine foot examinations in patients with diabetes in the primary care setting.[39]

Provider education as an intervention has not been studied as a preventive measure to decrease the incidence of foot ulcerations; however, several studies have revealed improvements in compliance with clinical practice recommendations as a result of clinician education. Interventions involving provider and clinical support staff education and feedback have shown to increase provider compliance with annual foot examination.[40] Clinical practice guidelines also have provided another avenue for education and reminders to practitioners regarding appropriate screening and management and have been found to increase compliance with recommended foot examinations for patients with diabetes.[41,42] Although provider education has been included as part of studies on complex or combined interventions for prevention of foot ulcers, this intervention has not been examined individually to assess the impact of this measure alone on the prevention of foot ulcers in patients with diabetes.

Skin Temperature Monitoring

Another recently investigated intervention for monitoring diabetic foot health and detecting areas at risk for development of diabetic foot ulcers is skin temperature monitoring. Various techniques currently are under investigation for this purpose, including electrical contact thermometry, cutaneous thermal discrimination thresholds, infrared thermometry, and liquid crystal thermography.[43] The theory behind this intervention is that pre-ulcerative inflammation can be detected as a relative elevation in skin temperature compared with the contralateral limb, and detection of an area at risk can prompt early intervention by the patient through modification of activity levels. In a single-blinded, randomized, controlled trial by Armstrong and colleagues, 225 patients were randomized to standard therapy alone (therapeutic footwear, diabetic foot education, regular foot care, and daily foot self-inspection) versus standard therapy with the addition of digital thermometry with infrared skin thermometers. Patients found to have temperature difference between limbs of 4° or more were asked to decrease activity levels until the temperature difference resolved. The thermometry group reported one-third the incidence of ulcers by the 18-month endpoint than patients in the standard treatment group.[44] Despite promising initial results, this technique has not yet been widely applied to clinical use.

Combined/Complex Interventions

Although specific interventions have been discussed independently in the interest of reviewing the current evidence regarding their efficacy, in practice, multiple interventions are often used simultaneously. Several studies have evaluated the effectiveness of these heterogeneous approaches to the care of feet of patients with diabetes. Many of these studies involve a tiered approach to intervention based on risk stratification of the patient.[45] Often, these complex interventions for at-risk patients take place in the setting of the specialized, multidisciplinary foot care clinics. Patient education and

Table 3
Complex interventions for prevention of ulceration

Author, Publication Year, Study Type	Population/ Stratification	Interventions	Outcome
Anichini, 2007, prospective cohort	1965 primary care patients with diabetes	Foot examination, screening for PVD and neuropathy by PCP; referral of high-risk patients to interdisciplinary foot care team	Decreased amputation rate 10.7–6.24/10 000 Decreased hospitalization rate
Lavery, 2005, prospective cohort	2738 HMO patients with diabetes	Provider education, foot examination, identification of risk factors for risk stratification Low risk: annual screening High risk: patient education, quarterly examination, orthotist examination and provision of shoes, insoles Ulcers: aggressive offloading, wound care, debridement, infection control, revascularization	47% decrease in amputation rate 37.8% decrease in foot-related hospitalization rate Hospital LOS decreased 21.7% SNF admission rate decreased 69.8% SNF LOS decreased 38.2%
Litzleman, 1993,[42] RCT	395 non-insulin-dependent patients with diabetes in primary care practice	Patient education Behavioral contract Provider education 12-month follow-up	Less serious foot lesions in intervention patients (rated by Seattle Wound Classification System) Intervention patients described better foot care behaviors Providers more likely to perform foot examinations

(continued on next page)

Table 3
(continued)

Author, Publication Year, Study Type	Population/ Stratification	Interventions	Outcome
Dargis, 1999, prospective cohort	145 patients with prior ulceration	Multidisciplinary clinic, foot care, education, specialized footwear, frequent foot care every 3 months	Reulceration rate:30% in intervention group, 58% control
Uccioli, 1995, RCT	69 patients with history of prior ulcer	Education, custom footwear, follow-up every 6 months Total follow-up 1 year	Reulceration: 27.7% intervention, 58.3 control
McCabe, 1998,[47,48] RCT	2001 patients from general diabetes clinic	Risk stratification, foot care, support hosiery, protective shoes, education	No significant difference in ulcerations Fewer major amputations
Patout, 2000, prospective cohort	197 patients with diabetes from low-income, African American population	Comprehensive foot clinic, interventions based on risk stratification Patient education, custom footwear, regular examinations	89% decrease in foot-related hospitalizations 49% decrease in days with open foot wound 79% decrease in lower extremity amputations

Abbreviations: RCT, randomized, controlled trial; SNF, skilled nursing facility.

Table 4
Interventions with evidence for decreasing the incidence of foot ulceration

Recommendation	Strength of Evidence	Comments
Offloading with foot orthotics for high-risk patients	A	Promotes resolution of callus May prevent reulceration in patients with prior history of foot ulcers
Patient education	A	Intensive educational sessions seem to decrease reulceration in patients with history of prior ulcer, amputation, or infection
Foot temperature monitoring	A	Limited studies of this intervention, not in widespread practice

Strength of evidence rating: A, randomized control trials and meta-analysis; B, other evidence, including well-designed controlled and uncontrolled studies.

routine foot examinations are generally included for patients in all categories in most of these interventional studies. Based on patient history and examination, patients deemed to be at higher risk for ulceration are generally followed with more frequent foot examinations and assessed for custom footwear if indicated.

Most complex intervention studies report decreased rates of ulceration, amputation, and hospitalization. Such an approach seems to be particularly effective in preventing ulceration in high-risk patients, such as those with a previous history of ulceration.[46] For example, Lavery and colleagues[45] implemented such a risk stratification program, with peripheral neuropathy as one deciding factor, to direct preventive interventions in a managed care organization and found that incidence of amputation decreased 47.4% and foot-related hospital admissions decreased 37.8% (**Table 3**).

COST-EFFECTIVENESS OF PREVENTION MEASURES

The financial impact of diabetic foot disease continues to grow in the United States and around the world. In 1 US-based observational cohort study performed over 2 years in a managed care institution, the attributable cost of care related to diabetic foot ulcer for the 2 years after diagnosis was approximately $28,000. Developing countries also may see the largest growth of cases of type 2 diabetes and subsequent complications over the next 20 years.[2] Several studies have examined the cost-effectiveness of interventions for the prevention of diabetic foot ulceration. In a cost-utility

Box 1
Interventions without adequate evidence for prevention of ulceration

Annual foot examination

Glycemic control

Medication

Revascularization

Provider education

Peripheral nerve decompression

analysis performed by Tennvall and Apelqvist in Sweden in 2001, preventive measures to decrease the incidence of ulceration (including podiatric foot examinations, specialty footwear, and patient education) were found to be cost-effective, assuming a decrease in the ulceration and amputation rate by 25%.[49] Another study by Ortegon and colleagues[50,51] in 2004 (Netherlands) also concluded that preventive measures of intensive glycemic control and optimal foot care were cost-effective, assuming a 40% risk reduction. Finally, the Centers for Disease Control and Prevention diabetes cost-effectiveness group concluded that intensive glycemic control is a cost-effective measure for reducing the risk of complications related to peripheral neuropathy and lower extremity amputations.[39]

SUMMARY

Foot ulceration in patients with diabetes is a costly and common problem and the leading cause of nontraumatic lower extremity amputation. With the rising global burden of diabetes in industrialized and developing nations, more attention is being dedicated to this issue. Although much effort has been put toward the study of treatment of ulcers, research on the prevention of this disease is still somewhat limited.

Multiple risk factors have been identified for ulceration and amputation. Those associated with risk of ulceration include peripheral neuropathy, history of prior ulceration or amputation, limited joint mobility, foot deformity, and abnormal foot pressures. Risk factors associated with amputation include peripheral vascular disease, peripheral neuropathy, lower extremity ulcers, former lower extremity amputation, and treatment with insulin. Evaluating patients for risk factors for ulceration or amputation may assist clinicians who are in risk stratification and public health organizations in allocating resources and targeting public health interventions toward patients most at risk. Interventions targeted at identifying patients at higher risk of ulceration and modification of risk factors have been found to decrease the incidence of hospital admission for diabetic foot wounds and lower extremity amputation. Specific interventions found to significantly decrease the incidence of diabetic foot ulcerations include offloading with foot orthotics for high-risk patients, patient education, complex/combined interventions and multidisciplinary approach, and foot temperature monitoring (**Table 4**).

Unfortunately, many of the current prevention interventions, such as annual foot examinations and glycemic control, have not proved to significantly decrease the incidence of ulceration. Other interventions, such as medications and revascularization, either have no significant evidence to support their usage or have not been studied adequately to make a determination regarding their utility toward this goal. Peripheral nerve decompression has been cited as a possible intervention to decrease the incidence of ulceration; however, reports are mixed on its effectiveness (**Box 1**).

REFERENCES

1. American Diabetes Association. Available at: www.diabetes.org. Accessed January 3, 2009.
2. Boulton AJM, Vilekyte L, Ragnarson-Tennvall, et al. The global burden of diabetic foot disease. Lancet 2005;366:1719–24.
3. International Working Group on the Diabetic Foot. Available at: www.iwgdf.org. Accessed 3 January, 2009.
4. Apelqvist J, Larsson J, Agardh CD. Long-term prognosis for diabetic patients with foot ulcers. J Intern Med 1993;233:485–91.
5. Centers for Disease Control and Prevention. Diabetes surveillance. Atlanta (GA): US Department of Health and Human Services; 1993. p. 87–93.

6. Cameron N, Cotter M, Inkster M, et al. Looking to the future: diabetic neuropathy and effects of rosuvastatin on neurovascular function in diabetes models. Diabetes Res Clin Pract 2003;61:S35–9.
7. Oyibo S, Jude EB, Tarawneh I. A comparison of two diabetic foot ulcer classification systems: the Wagner and University of Texas wound classification systems. Diabetes Care 2001;24:84–8.
8. Crawford F, Inkster M, Kleijnen J, et al. Predicting foot ulcers in patients with diabetes: a systematic review and meta-analysis. QJM 2007;100:65–86.
9. Frykberg RG, Lavery LA, Pham H, et al. Role of neuropathy and high foot pressures in diabetic foot ulceration. Diabetes Care 1998;21(10):1714–9.
10. Boyko EJ, Nelson KM, Ahroni JH, et al. Prediction of diabetic foot ulcer occurrence using commonly available clinical information. Diabetes Care 2006;29: 1202–7.
11. Reiber GE, Recoraro RE, Koepsell TD. Risk factors for amputation in patients with diabetes mellitus. Ann Intern Med 1992;117:97–105.
12. Adler AI, Ahroni JH, Boyko EJ, et al. Lower extremity amputation in diabetes: the independent effects of peripheral vascular disease, sensory neuropathy, and foot ulcers. Diabetes Care 1999;22(7):1029–35.
13. Sämann A, Tajiyeva O, Müller N, et al. Prevalence of the diabetic foot syndrome at the primary care level in Germany: a cross-sectional study. Diabet Med 2008;25: 557–63.
14. Stratton IM, Adler AI, Neil AW, et al. Association of glycaemia with macrovascular and microvascular complications of type 2 diabetes (UKPDS 35): prospective observational study. BMJ 2000;321:405–12.
15. The Diabetes Control and Complications Trial Research Group. The effect of intensive treatment of diabetes on the development and progression of long-term complications in insulin-dependent diabetes mellitus. N Engl J Med 1993; 329:977–86.
16. Steed DL, Attinger C, Brem H, et al. Guidelines for the prevention of diabetic ulcers. Wound Repair Regen 2008;16:169–74.
17. Caputo GM, Cavanagh PR, Ulbrech JS, et al. Assessment and management of foot disease in patients with diabetes. N Engl J Med 1994;331:854–60.
18. Armstrong DG, Lavery LA. Diabetic foot ulcers: prevention, diagnosis and classification. Am Fam Physician 1998;57(6):1325–32 1337–8.
19. O'Donnell ME, Badger SA, Anees Sharif M, et al. The effects of cilostazol on peripheral neuropathy in diabetic patients with peripheral arterial disease. Angiology 2009;59:695–704.
20. Gulcan E, Gulcan A, Erbilen E, et al. Statins may be useful in diabetic foot ulceration treatment and prevention. Med Hypotheses 2007;69:1313–5.
21. Emanueli C, Monopoli A, Kraenkel N, et al. Nitropravastatin stimulates reparative neovascularisation and improves recovery from limb ischaemia in type-1 diabetic mice. Br J Pharmacol 2007;150:873–82.
22. Chaudhry V, Russell J, Belzberg A. Decompressive surgery of lower limbs for symmetrical diabetic peripheral neuropathy. Cochrane Database Syst Rev 2008;(3):cd006152.
23. Aszmann O, Tassler PL, Dellon AL. Changing the natural history of diabetic neuropathy: incidence of ulcer/amputation in the contralateral limb of patients with a unilateral nerve decompression procedure. Ann Plast Surg 2004;53(6): 517–22.
24. American Diabetes Association. Preventive Foot Care in Diabetes. In: ADA position statement: preventative foot care. Diabetes Care 2004;27:S63–4.

25. Cowley MS, Boyko EJ, Shofer JB, et al. Foot ulcer risk and location in relation to prospective clinical assessment of foot shape and mobility among persons with diabetes. Diabetes Res Clin Pract 2008;82:226–32.
26. Mayfield JA, Reiber GE, Nelson RG, et al. Do foot examinations reduce the risk of diabetic amputation? J Fam Pract 2000;49:499–504.
27. Macfarlane RM, Jeffcoate WJ. Factors contributing to the presentation of diabetic foot ulcers. Diabet Med 1997;14:867–70.
28. Caselli A, Pham H, Giurini JM, et al. The forefoot-to-rearfoot plantar pressure ratio is increased in severe diabetic neuropathy and can predict foot ulceration. Diabetes Care 2002;6:1066–71.
29. Orlin MN, McPoil TG. Plantar pressure assessment. Phys Ther 2000;80:399–409.
30. Armstrong DG, Stacpoole-Shea S, Nguyen HC, et al. Lengthening of the Achilles tendon in diabetic patients who are at high risk for ulceration of the foot. J Bone Joint Surg Am 1999;81A:535–58.
31. Colagiuri S, Marsden LL, Naidu V, et al. Use of orthotic devices to correct plantar callus in people with diabetes. Diabetes Res Clin Pract 1995;28:29–34.
32. Bus SA, Valk GD, van Deursen RW, et al. The effectiveness of footwear and off-loading interventions to prevent and heal foot ulcers and reduce plantar pressures in diabetes: a systematic review. Diabetes Metab Res Rev 2008;24:S162–80.
33. Spencer SA. Pressure relieving interventions for preventing and treating diabetic foot ulcers. Cochrane Database Syst Rev 2000;(3):cd002302.
34. Uccioli L, Faglia E, Monticone G, et al. Manufactured shoes in the prevention of diabetic foot ulcers. Diabetes Care 1995;18(10):1376–8.
35. Busch K, Chantelau E. Effectiveness of a new brand of stock "diabetic" shoes to protect against diabetic foot ulcer relapse: a prospective cohort study. Diabet Med 2003;20:665–9.
36. Lincoln NB, Radford KA, Game FL, et al. Education for secondary prevention in people with diabetes: a randomized controlled trial. Diabetologia 2008;51:1954–61.
37. Valk GD, Kriegsman DMW, Assendelft WJJ. Patient education for preventing diabetic foot ulceration. Cochrane Database Syst Rev 2001;(4):cd001488.
38. American Diabetes Association. Preventive foot care in people with diabetes. Diabetes Care 2004;27:S63–4.
39. Wylie-Rosett J, Walker EA, Shamoon H, et al. Assessment of documented foot examinations for patients with diabetes in inner-city primary care clinics. Arch Fam Med 1995;4:46–50.
40. Kirkman MS, Williams SR, Caffrey HH, et al. Impact of a program to improve adherence to diabetes guidelines by primary care physicians. Diabetes Care 2002;25:1946–51.
41. Singh N, Armstrong DA, Lipsky BA. Preventing foot ulcers in patients with diabetes. JAMA 2005;293:217–28.
42. Litzelman DK, Slemenda CW, Langefeld CD, et al. Reduction of lower extremity clinical abnormalities in patients with non insulin-dependent diabetes mellitus. Ann Intern Med 1993;119:36–41.
43. Bharara M, Cobb JE, Claremont DJ. Thermography and thermometry in the assessment of diabetic neuropathic foot: a case for furthering the role of thermal techniques. Int J Low Extrem Wounds 2006;5(4):250–60.
44. Armstrong DG, Holtz-Neiderer K, Wendel C, et al. Skin temperature monitoring reduces the risk for diabetic foot ulceration in high-risk patients. Am J Med 2007;120:1042–6.

45. Lavery LA, Wunderlich RP, Tredwell JL. Disease management for the diabetic foot: effectiveness of a diabetic foot prevention program to reduce amputations and hospitalizations. Diabetes Res Clin Pract 2005;70:31–7.
46. Dargis V, Vileikyte L, Pantelejeva O, et al. Benefits of a multidisciplinary approach in the management of recurrent diabetic foot ulceration in Lithuania. Diabetes Care 1999;22:1428–31.
47. McCabe CJ, Stevenson RC, Dolan AM. Evaluation of a diabetic foot screening and protection program. Diabet Med 1998;15:80–4.
48. Ramsey SD, Newton K, Blough D. Incidence, outcomes, and cost of foot ulcers in patients with diabetes. Diabetes Care 1999;22:382–7.
49. Tennvall GR, Apelqvist J. Prevention of diabetes-related foot ulcers and amputations: a cost-utility analysis based on Markov model simulations. Diabetologia 2001;44:2077–87.
50. Ortegon MM, Redekop WK, Niessen LW. Cost-effectiveness of prevention and treatment of the diabetic foot: a Markov analysis. Diabetes Care 2004;27(4): 901–7.
51. The CDC Diabetes Cost-Effectiveness Group. Cost-effectiveness of intensive glycemic control, intensified hypertension control, and serum cholesterol level reduction for type 2 diabetes. JAMA 2002;287(19):2542–51.

Update in Diagnosis and Treatment of Diabetic Foot Infections

Andy O. Miller, MD*, Michael Henry, MD

KEYWORDS

- Diabetic foot ulcer • Diabetic foot infection • Review
- Osteomyelitis • Diabetes • Antibiotics

Foot infections rank high among the most feared and costly complications of diabetes mellitus. Levin and O'Neal[1] point out that there are 21 million diabetics, 42 million diabetic feet, and 210 million diabetic toes in the United States, minus the amputated ones. In the United States, it is estimated that perhaps 5% to 10% of diabetics sustain foot infections each year.[2] Diabetics have a 9- and 12-fold higher risk than their nondiabetic counterparts for developing cellulitis and osteomyelitis (OM) of the lower extremity, respectively.[3] Annually an estimated 82,000 limbs are lost as a result of diabetes.[4] Most diabetic foot infections (DFIs) are superficial; infection of deeper tissues occurs in about 25% of cases.[2,5] It is estimated that 25% to 50% of all DFIs require minor amputation, whereas 10% to 40% require major amputation. Sixty percent of all amputations in diabetics are preceded by an infected foot ulcer.[6,7] There is an increase in costs to patients, providers, and payers; of particular concern in at least 40% of patients undergoing major amputations is the loss in ability to live independently.[8]

Diabetic patients have many risk factors predisposing toward foot ulceration and infection, including previous amputations, peripheral sensorimotor and autonomic neuropathies, resultant osteoarthropathy, abnormal biomechanical stressors, vascular insufficiency, wound healing deficits, and reduced mobility and vision.[9] The impairment of neutrophil function in hyperglycemia and local hypoxic states also plays a major role. In 1 large cohort, independent clinical risk factors for the presence of infection in a diabetic foot ulcer (DFU) included penetration to bone, prior trauma, recurrent infection, duration of infection more than 30 days, and presence of

No funding source to be acknowledged.

Division of Infectious Diseases, Department of Medicine, Bronx-Lebanon Hospital Center, 1650 Grand Concourse, Bronx, NY 10457, USA

* Corresponding author.

E-mail address: amiller@bronxleb.org (A.O. Miller).

Phys Med Rehabil Clin N Am 20 (2009) 611–625
doi:10.1016/j.pmr.2009.06.007   pmr.theclinics.com

peripheral vascular disease.[2] Deep, recurrent, and multiple wounds are independently associated with development of OM.[10] A wide variety of modalities for diagnosis and treatment are available, with variable amounts of data supporting their use. The authors attempt to review salient recent data regarding diagnosis and treatment of DFIs. It is important to note that not all ulcers represent infections, although the vast majority of DFIs originate from DFUs. Studies vary greatly in the definition of "cure," but in general an infection may be "cured" without resolution of the underlying ulcer.

It should be noted that uninfected DFUs do not require antibiotic treatment. Multiple studies have considered the use of skin grafting, surgery, epidermal growth factors, hyperbaric oxygen, vacuum dressings, and other modalities for uninfected DFU therapy; treatment of these lesions is beyond the scope of this article.

PUBLISHED GUIDELINES

The Infectious Diseases Society of America (IDSA) issued extensive guidelines for the evaluation and treatment of DFIs in 2004.[11] An update is now nearing completion; the interested reader should refer to this work for updated recommendations. The IDSA guidelines, which are accessible at http://www.journals.uchicago.edu/doi/pdf/10.1086/424846, are recommended for their straightforward and pragmatic presentation of these complex issues. The International Working Group on the Diabetic Foot (IWGDF) published a similar set of guidelines in 2007 accessible at http://www.iwgdf.org/index.php and a recent set of proposed guidelines specifically for diabetic foot osteomyelitis (DFO).[12]

DIAGNOSING INFECTION
Initial Assessment

Despite the lack of clear consensus on numerous specific aspects of care for DFI, a general approach to care is commonly agreed upon. DFI must be diagnosed clinically and not based on the results of surface swab cultures. Signs of inflammation (local or systemic) in the presence of a DFU may suggest infection, although fever, leukocytosis, and elevated erythrocyte sedimentation rate (ESR) are present in less than 50% of cases.[13–15]

The initial clinical evaluation of DFI, as suggested in the 2004 IDSA guidelines, mandates evaluation of the overall physiologic and psychosocial state of the patient, the biomechanical and neurovascular status of the affected limb, and the detailed anatomy of the ulcer itself (**Table 1**).[11] The infected area should be assessed for extent of local necrosis, presence of abscesses, and possible involvement of bone or joints.

After establishing the presence of a DFI, the patient should first be assessed for the presence of any signs of systemic response to infection, as well as the metabolic state. This will help triage the patient, helping the clinician determine the level of urgency required in addressing the infection, and determining the best venue for care. On presentation, the wound should be specifically assessed for the severity and extent of the infection.

The severity of a DFI dictates the initial course of treatment, including selection of antibiotic, route of administration, and duration of treatment, as well as the need for hospitalization. The IDSA and the IWGDF guidelines present similar classification schemes of infection severity (**Table 2**).[16] These schemes were recently validated in a longitudinal study of 1666 diabetic patients, which found that with an increasing class of severity, there was a significantly increased risk for amputation, higher-level amputation, and lower-extremity hospitalization.[16]

Table 1
Initial assessment of a patient with a DFI

Level of Evaluation	Relevant Problems and Observations	Investigations
Patient		
Systemic response to inflammation	Fevers, chills, sweats, vomiting, hypotension, tachycardia	History and physical examination
Metabolic state	Volume depletion, azotemia, hyperglycemia, tachypnea, hyperosmolality, acidosis	Serum chemistry analyses and hematologic testing
Cognitive state	Delirium, dementia, depression	Assessment of mental status
Social situation	Self-neglect, noncompliance, lack of home support	Interviews with family, friends, health care professionals
Limb or foot		
Biomechanics	Deformities (Charcot, claw/hammer toes, calluses)	Clinical examination and radiography (≥ 2 images)
Vascular Status		
Arterial	Ischemia, necrosis, gangrene	Foot pulses, ABI, TcPo$_2$, duplex ultrasonography, angiography
Venous	Edema, stasis, or thrombosis	Physical examination and duplex ultrasonography
Neuropathy	Loss of protective sensation	Light touch, microfilament pressure, or vibration perception
Wound		
Size and depth (tissues involved)	Necrosis, gangrene, foreign body, and involvement of deeper tissues	Inspect, debride, and probe the wound; radiography (≥ 2 images)
Presence, extent, and cause of infection	Purulence, warmth, tenderness, pain, induration, cellulites, bullae, crepitus, abscess, fasciitis, and osteomyelitis	Gram stain, culture of deep tissue, imaging (see text)

OM is often missed in the absence of inflammatory signs, but is present in approximately 20% of all DFI and complicates its management more than any other single factor.[12] Acute Charcot arthropathy or gout is a noninfectious cause of foot inflammation that can mimic DFO. OM serves as a very poor prognostic marker, greatly increasing the likelihood that the patient will ultimately require amputation. In the rest of this article, the management of diabetic foot complicated by OM is discussed separately from soft-tissue DFIs.

Microbiology of the Diabetic Foot

As opposed to normally sterile body sites (bladder, CNS, intravascular space), ulcerated and normal skin are colonized by a varied range of microorganisms, of which a limited set (eg, gram-positive cocci such as *Staphylococcus aureus* and Group B

Table 2
Comparison of DFI severity classification schemes

Clinical Description	IDSA	IWDGF
Wound without purulence or any manifestations of inflammation	Uninfected	1
≥2 Manifestations of inflammation (purulence or erythema, pain, tenderness, warmth, or induration); any cellulitis or erythema extends ≥2 cm around ulcer, and infection is limited to skin or superficial subcutaneous tissues; no local complications or systemic illness	Mild	2
Infection in a patient who is systemically well and metabolically stable but has ≥1 of the following: cellulitis extending 12 cm; lymphangitis; spread beneath fascia; deep tissue abscess; gangrene; muscle, tendon, joint, or bone involvement	Moderate	3
Infection in a patient with systemic toxicity or metabolic instability (eg, fever, chills, tachycardia, hypotension, confusion, vomiting, leukocytosis, acidosis, hyperglycemia, or azotemia)	Severe	4

streptococci, and gram-negative bacilli such as *Klebsiella* and *Pseudomonas)* can act as pathogens. Although newer molecular methods show the diversity of fastidious flora in most DFI,[17] the clinical utility of identifying such organisms is not clear. Normal skin, as opposed to ulcerated skin, has an ability to limit the residence and invasion of common skin pathogens. Infection is distinguished from colonization of such tissue by the presence of local tissue destruction and inflammation—not by the presence or absence of pathogenic bacteria.

Pathogens causing DFIs and OM are the same, although *S. aureus* is proportionally overrepresented in OM (in 1 study, *S. aureus* 40%, Enterobacteriaceae such as *Escherichia coli* or *Klebsiella pneumoniae* 40%, streptococci 30%, *S. epidermidis* 25%).[18] Specific syndromes associated with particular bacteria include macerated ulcers after soaking (*Pseudomonas*) and "fetid foot" (a gangrenous and/or necrotic malodorous foot as a result of mixed aerobic and/or anaerobic infection). More commonly, a patient will present with a DFI that is antibiotic-naïve (wherein gram-positive organisms predominate) or previously treated (wherein resistant gram-negative bacteria become likelier, with increased antibiotic resistance seen after broader and longer courses of antibiotics).[11] Among the few published cases of fully vancomycin-resistant *S. aureus* (VRSA), dysvascular patients have been highly represented (so far, VRSA has been found in 1 diabetic foot[19]), highlighting the need for vigilance and antibiotic stewardship in DFI management.

Wound Cultures

A swab culture of the surface of a DFU usually reveals at least 1 potential pathogen; such surface cultures can be difficult to use in guiding treatment because they do not distinguish a colonized ulcer from an infected one. Culturing an uninfected DFU is rarely necessary (except in limited cases when screening for resistant colonizing flora). Swab cultures of the surface of an infected DFU often fail to represent the underlying pathogen.[20] When deep DFIs are suspected, deep cultures are most suitable for guiding antibiotic therapy.

In most cases, cultures of DFI should be obtained before the start of treatment (although a recent study found a striking lack of association between receipt of prior antibiotics and bone culture positivity).[21] When cultures are obtained, the technique used to obtain tissue for culture and the type of tissue taken strongly affect the validity of the result. Ideally, deep cultures should be obtained without traversing the wound bed, to avoid the potential contamination of deep tissue with surface colonizing flora. After removing overlying necrotic debris, specimens should be obtained from the wound base or deeper tissues. It is important not to rely upon cultures from undebrided wounds or from wound drainage, whose correlation with deep cultures is poor. Blood cultures should be obtained in systemically ill patients. Aerobic and anaerobic bacterial cultures are sufficient in most cases to yield a diagnosis; fungi, mycobacteria, and viruses are uncommon causes of DFI.

New molecular methods attempt to determine whether cultured isolates are colonizers or pathogens by identifying specific virulence factors.[22] Although these strategies are intriguing, their clinical utility remains unproven at this point.

Diagnosis of Diabetic Foot Osteomyelitis

In many cases of DFI, presence of infection is evident but severity and extent are not **(Fig. 1)**. The need for surgery, the duration of antibiotics, and the outcome all depend strongly on whether the underlying pedal bone is infected. Because diabetic peripheral neuropathy predisposes to Charcot disease, which can mimic OM, distinction of infected and uninfected bone is usually difficult.

Physical examination
Physical examination plays a key role in the assessment of OM in DFI. DFO is typically defined as contiguous spread of infection from the soft tissue to bone, through the cortex, into the marrow space. The possibility of OM should be considered in all DFU, but particularly in larger (>2 cm), deeper (>3 mm), and more chronic ulcers. Swollen ("sausage") toes and elevated ESR further suggest OM.[23–25] The probe-to-bone test has a high positive predictive value in patients with suspected DFO. When exposed bone is observed, or a metal probe advanced into the ulcer comes in contact with bone (where it produces a characteristic feel), OM is likely (sensitivity 60%, specificity 91%).[26,27]

Laboratory testing
Leukocytosis is generally a poor marker for OM.[14] ESR and C-reactive protein tests on their own are inadequate to diagnose OM, but when coupled with clinical assessments (ie, ulcer size) their utility is somewhat augmented.[28]

Imaging for osteomyelitis
Plain x-rays should be ordered for most patients with a DFU,[11] despite sensitivity for DFO around 54%.[27] Observable radiographic changes generally do not occur in the first 2 weeks of OM, which may explain in part the lack of sensitivity observed in clinical studies. Early changes classically seen in OM on x-ray imaging include periosteal reaction, focal osteopenia, or erosions; sequestrum, or islands of necrosed bone, can be seen in later chronic OM. Because the sensitivity of x-rays increases substantially with time, stable patients with suspected OM and negative initial plain films can be reimaged 2 weeks later.[11]

Advanced imaging
Studies of advanced imaging techniques in diagnosing DFO have variable results; as a general observation higher pretest likelihoods of OM enhance the evaluated performance characteristics of these tests.[29] Bone scans are reasonably sensitive (approximately 80%–85%) but nonspecific (approximately 30%–40%).[27] Indium-111–tagged

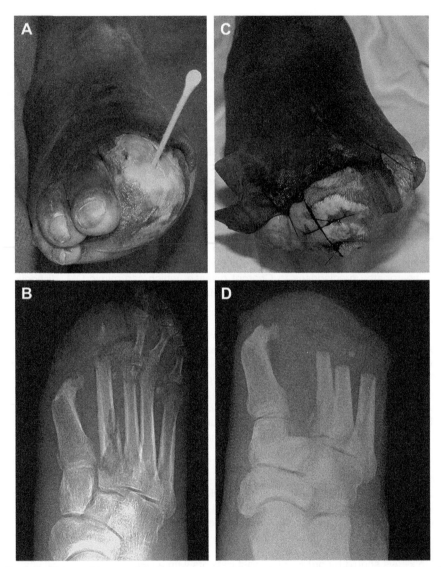

Fig. 1. A 47-year-old man with diabetes and peripheral neuropathy with gas gangrene of forefoot after auto-amputation of hallux and second toe. (*A*) Preoperative image illustrating deep space infection through purulent stump wound. Cotton tip applicator probing deeply to bone shows depth of infection. (*B*) Preoperative radiographs with subcutaneous gas and obvious osteomyelitic destruction of the entire second metatarsal, third metatarsal head and neck, and fourth metatarsophalangeal joint. (*C & D*) Postoperative photograph and radiograph (postop day 1) after incision and drainage, transmetatarsal amputation, and resection of entire second metatarsal for infection. Intraoperative bone culture grew *Proteus mirabilis*. (*Courtesy of* Neal Blitz, DPM, FACFAS, Bronx, NY.)

leukocyte scans offer somewhat improved specificity (75%). Other radiolabeling techniques include sulesomab and Tc-dextran scintigraphy[30,31] which have yet to become common. High-resolution ultrasound and PET scanning also show promise, but few data are available.[32]

Magnetic resonance imaging (MRI) is the imaging procedure of choice when OM is suspected, but not confirmed, by initial examination. MRI offers superior sensitivity and specificity (approximately 90% and 80%, respectively).[27] Defects in soft tissue can be visualized along with infected bone. MRI-based diagnosis of OM can be confounded by false positive results (from Charcot disease) or false negative results (in early OM).

Bone biopsy

In contrast to laboratory and radiologic testing, bone biopsy provides a definitive diagnosis of OM. Studies of DFO[20,33–36] and other types of chronic lower extremity OM[37] convincingly show the limitations of shallow cultures for the identification of deep pathogens. The oft-cited caveat to this recommendation is the presence of a monomicrobial *S. aureus* culture from a draining sinus, which correlates highly with the presence of *S. aureus* in the bone culture.[38]

Bone biopsies should be performed without traversing the open ulcer, using surgical or interventional radiographic approaches, to avoid contamination with surface flora. Open bone biopsies during surgery or debridement are more easily obtained, but may be more commonly contaminated by ulcer microflora.[20]

Bone biopsy specimens should be sent for histopathology and bacterial culture (both aerobic and anaerobic). Histopathology can show osteitis or osteonecrosis that provide a definitive diagnosis. A positive culture result provides an opportunity for targeted antibiotic selection, with resultant decreases in the risk for adverse events, selection of resistant flora, and cost. Bone biopsy is most useful in cases where the diagnosis remains in question, or when the patient's previous culture results or antibiotic therapy require a specific microbiologic diagnosis.

Treatment

General approach

In principle, the treatment of a diabetic foot seems to be straightforward, with clear goals: stabilization of the patient, control of the infection, prevention of infection-related morbidities, and preservation of function. An initial treatment plan of a DFI is often a 2-pronged attack of antibiotic therapy and surgical intervention of varying intensity; and it includes decisions regarding wound dressing, off-loading, and close, systematic follow-up by a multidisciplinary team, which includes infectious disease specialists, surgeons, endocrinologists, podiatrists, and physiatrists.[11] Unfortunately, the optimal approach to many aspects remains unclear, in spite of innumerable studies focusing on the care of DFIs.

Factors complicating the establishment of an optimal approach

The treatment of DFIs has been the subject of countless clinical trials and publications over the past decades. Despite the surfeit of data, the goal of establishing an optimal, evidenced-based approach to the management of this problem remains beyond reach. Several factors contribute to this situation. The vast majority of clinical trials have been noncomparative and nonrandomized. The terms used in recent history to describe DFI severity, extent, and outcome have not been standardized. There is little agreement as to what even constitutes an important outcome measure. Thus drawing meaningful conclusions from the collective experience represented in the literature proves challenging.

Compounding these issues is the fact that, when controlled clinical trials have been conducted, many of the attempts at designing them have been hampered by small size, poor design, and lack of replication. Underscoring this problem is a recent systematic review of controlled clinical trials assessing antimicrobial interventions for DFUs. Of 1903 identified trials, only 23 were deemed to be of sufficient quality to contribute meaningful results.[39]

Venue of treatment

One of the first decisions faced by the clinician treating a diabetic wound infection is determining if hospitalization is required. In most instances, patients with mild infections can be treated in the outpatient setting with oral antibiotics and close clinical follow-up.[40] Very few studies have assessed the efficacy of outpatient antibiotic management of DFIs. The largest such study was an Italian multicenter observation trial of 271 patients treated for DFIs in the outpatient setting.[41] A cure or improvement was documented in 93.4% of those enrolled, reflecting the results of previous smaller studies. Of note, approximately 60% of the patients in this study received parenteral outpatient antibiotics.

Patients who meet the criteria for severe infections almost always require hospitalization. Moderate DFI cases need to be assessed on a case-by-case basis; in the absence of complicating features, these patients can generally be treated as outpatients.[11] However, a number of factors need to be considered, including the management of metabolic instability and pain. Often, hospitalization is prompted by the need for diagnostic tests or intravenous antibiotics when they cannot be arranged on an outpatient basis in a timely manner. The complexity of dressing changes and the ability of a patient to comply with treatment also need to be assessed when considering the need for admission.

Antibiotic choice

There is little evidence from randomized clinical trials to guide antibiotic selection or duration. There is even controversy over which bacteria cultured from the wound require specific treatment.[12] No specific regimen has found to be more effective than others.[39,42] Many different antibiotics have the potential to treat most common bacteria that cause DFIs. Therefore, an appropriate empiric regimen must be selected from an array of antibiotics, guided by clinical severity and local antibiotic resistance patterns.[11,43] There is little evidence to suggest that targeting all isolated pathogens in a polymicrobial culture is necessary. This point is underscored by the results of several recent studies evaluating newer agents in the treatment of DFIs. Monotherapy with relatively narrower-spectrum antibiotics (linezolid, daptomycin, ertapenem, and moxifloxacin) was equivalent to monotherapy with broader-spectrum comparator antibiotics, even when organisms resistant to the antibiotic regimen were isolated.[44–46]

Despite the lack of a preferred regimen for DFIs, treatment guidelines agree that targeting S. aureus is paramount. S. aureus is the most common cause of DFI, and empiric antibiotic coverage should always include an antistaphylococcal agent.[11] In the absence of risk factors for methicillin-resistant S. aureus (MRSA), the frequent use of first generation cephalosporins and antistaphylococcal penicillins needs to be assessed carefully.[47] Nevertheless, it is interesting to note that 2 large, well-conducted randomized controlled trials found that in patients with polymicrobial wound infections containing MRSA, receipt of vancomycin was not associated with a change in clinical outcome.[44,45] Despite these findings, MRSA should not be ignored when isolated from a DFI; rather these findings again show the difficulty in determining the pathogenic role of specific organisms. In general, less virulent gram-positive organisms (coagulase-negative staphylococci and diphtheroid species) do not need to be directly treated. Enterococcus, another gram-positive organism, does not typically require targeted therapy when isolated in polymicrobial infection.[44,46]

Empiric treatment of aerobic gram-negative organisms (ie, *K. pneumoniae*, *E. coli*, and *Proteus* species) should be restricted to patients presenting with severe DFI or those with chronically infected diabetic wounds with prior antibiotic exposure.[11] The specter of *Pseudomonas* looms large when selecting an empiric regimen of antibiotics for moderate to severe DFIs. Determining when to target *Pseudomonas* remains unclear. It is commonly found as part of a polymicrobial infection, but its role as a pathogen in this setting is difficult to determine. Some experts suggest that treatment does not need to be directed at *Pseudomonas* unless it is the predominant organism isolated from a deep tissue specimen, or if the patient presents with sepsis.[42] The growing prevalence of extended spectrum beta-lactamase *E. coli* and *K. pneumoniae* in DFIs is of great concern. As these organisms become more common, the approach to empiric antibiotic therapy for DFIs will become increasingly complicated.[43]

This difficulty in deciding whether to target a cultured organism also clouds the treatment of obligate anaerobes, like peptococci, peptostreptococci, and *Bacteroides* species. These organisms, too, can often be isolated from polymicrobial infections; their overall contribution to the infection is likely to be minimal. Only when there is severe necrosis or gangrene do obligate anaerobes need to be specifically targeted.[46]

Duration and route of therapy

As with choice of antibiotics, the duration of therapy for DFIs has not been systematically studied. Current guidelines suggests that 1 to 2 weeks of oral therapy are adequate for mild DFI, whereas 2 to 4 weeks of oral therapy should be administered for moderate and severe cases as long as there is no associated OM.[11,40] The approach to DFO is discussed in the following section.

In spite of these seemingly clear recommendations, it is often difficult and possibly risky to determine a priori the exact duration of treatment. The optimal length of antibiotic therapy in a given individual is dependent on a substantial range of variables. Removal of necrotic tissue and pus, and selection of antibiotics with advantageous pharmacokinetics, can significantly reduce the total duration of antibiotics required. Antibiotic concentrations achieved in the infected tissue may affect outcome. Common sense suggests that in a patient with a severely impaired vascular supply to the infected foot, the ability of antibiotics to reach their target will be hindered. Most studies evaluating this scenario have been small; some report decreased levels of antibiotics in ischemic tissues despite adequate serum levels, but others have found the opposite.[48,49]

The need for flexibility and common sense in deciding whether to stop or continue antibiotic therapy is emphasized in the existing guidelines. Both sets of guidelines present algorithms to assist clinicians with assessing for an inadequate response to treatment. Ultimately, careful follow-up is essential in determining when to stop antibiotics.

Topical antibiotics

Topical local administration of antimicrobials to DFI has several potential advantages, such as increased target site concentration, avoidance of systemic toxicity, and preservation of normal bowel flora. In addition, some potentially effective agents (ie, mupirocin, pexiganan) can only be administered topically. Regardless of their benefits, the role of topical antimicrobial or antiseptic therapy is limited to mild infection; these agents do not penetrate tissue far beyond their site of application and are therefore inappropriate for deeper infection. Certain topical agents may in fact inhibit wound healing on a cellular level.[46]

Until very recently, no topical agent had been shown to be effective in any clinical trials.[39] In 2008, a randomized controlled trial of more than 800 patients evaluated the efficacy of pexiganan, an antimicrobial peptide, in comparison to ofloxacin for the treatment of mildly infected DFIs. It showed equivalent outcomes in regards to overall clinical improvement, microbiological eradication rates, and wound healing rates.[50]

Determination of the need for surgery

The role of surgery in DFIs is dual: the first goal is to control deep infection and the second is to salvage the foot. Many DFIs present with an obvious need for surgical intervention, ranging from simple debridement to emergent amputation in the setting of critical limb ischemia or necrotizing fasciitis. A systemically ill patient may not respond positively despite appropriate antibiotics until the infection has been adequately debrided.[5]

Despite the many obvious benefits of surgical intervention, increased risk for morbidity may exist. Deformities created by surgery can have deleterious long-term effects on wound healing as well as the function of the limb.[51] A surgeon must consider the blood supply to the remaining tissue, the effect of the proposed surgery on biomechanical function, and the optimal approach to wound closure.

Early surgical intervention has been shown to decrease the need for eventual amputation, decrease the time needed for return to function, and to reduce the duration of antibiotics.[52] Patients with noncritical ischemia can generally be treated without revascularization. In the setting of critical ischemia, early revascularization (within 24–48 hours) is advisable to avoid amputation[53] although sepsis may lead to unavoidable delays. However, much like the evidence guiding antibiotic management, the body of literature pertaining to the best surgical approach to DFIs is lacking in consistent conclusions.[11,54] Comparative and randomized studies of surgical treatment, using consistent terminology and techniques, are lacking.[55,56] Although the benefits of surgery in the short-term can be self-evident, very few studies have reported the long-term outcome of surgery in the infected diabetic foot.[51]

Diabetic foot osteomyelitis

The approach to management of DFO is highly controversial. Despite the frequent occurrence and high morbidity of DFO, published literature provides little guidance as to the optimal approach to treatment.[12,21] It is important to understand that DFO is generally a result of contiguous spread of infection from overlying tissue. Often, the presence of OM can be difficult to detect clinically.[38] As a result DFO is typically chronic when it is finally identified.[21] Unlike acute hematogenous OM, for which a 4- to 6-week course of antibiotics is typically curative, chronic OM (in nondiabetics as well as diabetics) has historically required antibiotics and surgical debridement of devitalized bone.[11] Opinions vary on the necessity and timing of surgical treatment. Some studies recommend aggressive early surgery in almost every patient.[21,57] Conversely, a growing body of literature reports successful treatment with antibiotic therapy and surgical debridement in certain selected patients.[58,59] As a result, there is no clear standard of care for the management of DFO. Current guidelines allow that in some cases, antibiotic therapy alone can be sufficient to achieve cure in DFO, but predicting which patients will ultimately fail medical management cannot be done with any certainty.[11,12]

Several factors complicate the choice of antibiotics in DFO. Adequate antibiotic penetration of infected bone historically mandates the use of intravenous preparations, but the availability of several highly bioavailable oral antibiotics question the necessity of this practice.[56] Treatment duration in DFO is often long, increasing the risk for antibiotic-related side effects, but the optimal duration of antibiotic is not well understood. Although treating susceptible organisms with antibiotic monotherapy is usually sufficient, exceptions exist (ie, quinolones or rifampin as monotherapy for S. aureus). The IDSA guidelines suggest basing the duration on the extent of residual viable and necrotic tissue after debridement: if all necrotic tissue is successfully removed, treatment can be as short as 2 to 5 days. In the presence of residual infected or necrotic bone, there is no clear endpoint to antibiotic therapy.

Adjunctive modalities

Several other modalities have been employed to treat DFIs. These include negative-pressure wound healing (eg, V.A.C. dressings, KCI, San Antonio, TX, USA), hyperbaric oxygen therapy, granulocyte colony stimulating factor (GCSF), and maggot debridement therapy (MDT). These modalities have most often been studied in noninfected DFU, or in some cases in DFI following surgery. As is the case with most aspects of diabetic foot management, case series and anecdotal reports comprise most of the current body of evidence evaluating these treatments; definitive evidence for their efficacy is lacking. The IDSA guidelines do not address the use of these adjunctive therapies for DFIs. In the more specific setting of DFO, the IWGDF recommendations for DFO state simply "there is no evidence to support the use of hyperbaric oxygen, granulocyte colony stimulating factor (G-CSF) or larval therapy in the treatment of diabetic foot osteomyelitis."[12] Negative-pressure wound healing is not addressed.

Negative-pressure wound healing was found to be most likely safe and beneficial in a subset of patients in a recent review of the few randomized controlled trials available.[60] In 2 of the larger studies evaluating any adjunctive therapy, benefit has been found in postsurgical patients recovering from a transmetatarsal amputation in the setting of DFO[61] and the treatment of noninfected diabetic wounds, as compared with standard wound dressing.[62] DFI not managed with transmetatarsal amputation has not been systematically studied.

Hyperbaric oxygen therapy was found to lead to a significant reduction in the need for major amputation and improved healing at 1 year in a recent systematic review. The number of patients enrolled in the available studies was small, however, and design flaws limited the studies' usefulness.[63]

A recent meta-analysis of GCSF therapy analyzed data from 167 patients and found a significant reduction in surgical intervention in the treatment arm, including amputations. There was also a tendency toward decreased antibiotic use.[64] Larger scale studies are required.

MDT is a simple, efficient method to separate necrotic tissue from living tissue, typically using larvae of the fly Lucilia sericata. It has been used in cases of DFI not responding to conventional therapy, but randomized controlled trials do not yet exist.[60,65]

Summary

A multidisciplinary approach to postinfection wound management, with off-loading, intensive rehabilitation, and a wound care program, improves outcomes.[11] Control of diabetes and vasculopathy is important to enhance wound healing and prevent recurrences. Treatment leads to a good clinical response in 80% to 90% of mild to moderate infections and 60% to 80% of deeper infections, including OM. Relapse occurs in 20% to 30% of cases, notably in those with OM or poor vascular supply.[11]

DFIs, a major cause of morbidity, mortality, and health care expenditure in diabetics, are common and frequently pose difficult diagnostic and therapeutic problems.

Although new studies slowly advance our knowledge of optimal therapy, the evidence base remains incomplete. Diagnosis requires careful physical examination, often coupled with data from radiology, microbiology, pathology, and the laboratory. A multidisciplinary approach with careful antibiotic selection, surgery in selected cases, and attention to physiologic and biomechanical parameters of healing remains the cornerstone of treatment. New techniques, and refinements of current methods, will lead to better care for these devastating and costly infections.

REFERENCES

1. Levin ME, O'Neal LW. Foreword. In: Bowker JH, Pfeifer MA, editors. Levin and O'Neal's the diabetic foot. 7th edition. Philadelphia: Mosby; 2008. p. xi–xiii.
2. Lavery LA, Armstrong DG, Wunderlich RP, et al. Risk factors for foot infections in individuals with diabetes. Diabetes Care 2006;29:1288–93.
3. Boyko EJ, Lipsky BA. Infection in diabetes mellitus. In: Harris MI, editor. Diabetes in America. 2nd edition. NIH publication No 95-1468. Bethesda (MD): National Institutes of Health; 1995. p. 485–99.
4. "Diabetes" International Diabetes Federation. Available at: http://www.idf.org/webdata/docs/background_info_NA.pdf. Accessed July 8, 2009.
5. Lipsky BA. Infectious problems of the foot in diabetic patients. In: Bowker JH, Pfeifer MA, editors. Levin and O'Neal's the diabetic foot. 7th edition. Philadelphia: Mosby; 2008. p. 305–18.
6. Pecoraro RE, Ahroni JH, Boyko EJ, et al. Chronology and determinants of tissue repair in diabetic lower-extremity ulcers. Diabetes 1991;40(10):1305–13.
7. Reiber GE, Pecoraro RE, Koepsell TD. Risk factors for amputation in patients with diabetes mellitus. A case-control study. Ann Intern Med 1992;117(2):97–105.
8. Larsson J, Agardh CD, Apelqvist J, et al. Long-term prognosis after healed amputation in patients with diabetes. Clin Orthop Relat Res 1998 May;(350):149–58.
9. Peters EJ, Lavery LA, Armstrong DG. Diabetic lower extremity infection: influence of physical, psychological, and social factors. J Diabetes Complications 2005; 19(2):107–12.
10. Lavery LA, Peters EJ, Armstrong DG, et al. Risk factors for developing osteomyelitis in patients with diabetic foot wounds. Diabetes Res Clin Pract 2009;83(3): 347–52.
11. Lipsky BA, Berendt AR, Deery HG, et al. Diagnosis and treatment of diabetic foot infections. Clin Infect Dis 2004;39:885–910.
12. Berendt AR, Peters EJ, Bakker K, et al. Diabetic foot osteomyelitis: a progress report on diagnosis and a systematic review of treatment. Diabetes Metab Res Rev 2008;24(Suppl 1):S145–61.
13. Eneroth M, Apelqvist J, Stenström A. Clinical characteristics and outcome in 223 diabetic patients with deep foot infections. Foot Ankle Int 1997;18(11):716–22.
14. Armstrong DG, Lavery LA, Sariaya M, et al. Leukocytosis is a poor indicator of acute osteomyelitis of the foot in diabetes mellitus. J Foot Ankle Surg 1996; 35(4):280–3, 14–43.
15. Armstrong DG, Perales TA, Murff RT, et al. Value of white blood cell count with differential in the acute diabetic foot infection. J Am Podiatr Med Assoc 1996; 86(5):224–7, 14–45.
16. Lavery LA, Armstrong DG, Murdoch DP, et al. Validation of the Infectious Diseases Society of America's diabetic foot infection classification system. Clin Infect Dis 2007;44:562–5.

17. Dowd SE, Wolcott RD, Sun Y, et al. Polymicrobial nature of chronic diabetic foot ulcer biofilm infections determined using bacterial tag encoded FLX amplicon pyrosequencing (bTEFAP). PLoS ONE 2008;3(10):e3326.
18. Lipsky BA. Osteomyelitis of the foot in diabetic patients. Clin Infect Dis 1997; 25(6):1318–26, 14–59.
19. CDC. Vancomycin-resistant *Staphylococcus aureus*—Pennsylvania, 2002. MMWR Morb Mortal Wkly Rep 2002;51:902.
20. Senneville E, Melliez H, Beltrand E, et al. Culture of percutaneous bone biopsy specimens for diagnosis of diabetic foot osteomyelitis: concordance with ulcer swab cultures. Clin Infect Dis 2006;42:57–62.
21. Aragón-Sánchez FJ, Cabrera-Galván JJ, Quintana-Marrero Y, et al. Outcomes of surgical treatment of diabetic foot osteomyelitis: a series of 185 patients with histopathological confirmation of bone involvement. Diabetologia 2008;51(11): 1962–70.
22. Sotto A, Lina G, Richard JL, et al. Virulence potential of Staphylococcus aureus strains isolated from diabetic foot ulcers: a new paradigm. Diabetes Care 2008;31:2318–24.
23. Rajbhandari SM, Sutton M, Davies C, et al. 'Sausage toe': a reliable sign of underlying osteomyelitis. Diabet Med 2000;17(1):74–7.
24. Kaleta JL, Fleischli JW, Reilly CH. The diagnosis of osteomyelitis in diabetes using erythrocyte sedimentation rate: a pilot study. J Am Podiatr Med Assoc 2001; 91(9):445–50.
25. Karr JC. The diagnosis of osteomyelitis in diabetes using erythrocyte sedimentation rate. J Am Podiatr Med Assoc 2002;92(5):314 [author reply 314–5].
26. Grayson ML, Gibbons GW, Balogh K, et al. Probing to bone in infected pedal ulcers. A clinical sign of underlying osteomyelitis in diabetic patients. JAMA 1995;273(9):721–3.
27. Dinh MT, Abad CL, Safdar N. Diagnostic accuracy of the physical examination and imaging tests for osteomyelitis underlying diabetic foot ulcers: meta-analysis. Clin Infect Dis 2008;47(4):519–27.
28. Fleischer AE, Didyk AA, Woods JB, et al. Combined clinical and laboratory testing improves diagnostic accuracy for osteomyelitis in the diabetic foot. J Foot Ankle Surg 2009;48:39–46.
29. Wrobel JS, Connolly JE. Making the diagnosis of osteomyelitis. The role of prevalence. J Am Podiatr Med Assoc 1998;88(7):337–43.
30. Delcourt A, Huglo D, Prangere T, et al. Comparison between Leukoscan (Sulesomab) and Gallium-67 for the diagnosis of osteomyelitis in the diabetic foot. Diabetes Metab 2005;31(2):125–33.
31. Sarikaya A, Aygit AC, Pekindil G. Utility of 99mTc dextran scintigraphy in diabetic patients with suspected osteomyelitis of the foot. Ann Nucl Med 2003;17(8): 669–76.
32. Keidar Z, Militianu D, Melamed E, et al. The diabetic foot: initial experience with 18F-FDG PET/CT. J Nucl Med 2005;46(3):444–9.
33. Khatri G, Wagner DK, Sohnle PG. Effect of bone biopsy in guiding antimicrobial therapy for osteomyelitis complicating open wounds. Am J Med Sci 2001;321(6): 367–71.
34. Zuluaga AF, Galvis W, Saldarriaga JG, et al. Etiologic diagnosis of chronic osteomyelitis: a prospective study. Arch Intern Med 2006;166(1):95–100.
35. Kessler L, Piemont Y, Ortega F, et al. Comparison of microbiological results of needle puncture vs. superficial swab in infected diabetic foot ulcer with osteomyelitis. Diabet Med 2006;23(1):99–102.

36. Zuluaga AF, Galvis W, Jaimes F, et al. Lack of microbiological concordance between bone and non-bone specimens in chronic osteomyelitis: an observational study. BMC Infect Dis 2002;2:8.
37. Mackowiak PA, Jones SR, Smith JW. Diagnostic value of sinus-tract cultures in chronic osteomyelitis. JAMA 1978;239(26):2772–5.
38. Johnston B, Conly J. Osteomyelitis management: more art than science? Can J Infect Dis Med Microbiol 2007;18:115–8.
39. Nelson EA, O'Meara S, Golder S, et al. Systematic review of antimicrobial treatments for diabetic foot ulcers. Diabetic Medicine 2006;23:348–59.
40. Lipsky BA, Pecoraro RE, Larson SA, et al. Outpatient management of uncomplicated lower-extremity infections in diabetic patients. Arch Intern Med 1990;150:790–7.
41. Esposito S, Leone S, Noviello S, et al. Foot infections in diabetes (DFIs) in the outpatient setting: an Italian multicentre observational survey. Diabetic Med 2008;25:979–84.
42. Lipsky BA. Empirical therapy for diabetic foot infections: are there clinical clues to guide antibiotic selection? Clin Microbiol Infect 2007;13:351–3.
43. Khanolkar MP, Bain SC, Stephens JW. The diabetic foot. QJM 2008;101:685–95.
44. Lipsky BA, Armstrong DG, Citron DM, et al. Ertapenem versus piperacillin/tazobactam for diabetic foot infections (SIDESTEP): prospective, randomised, controlled, double-blinded, multicentre trial. Lancet 2005;366:1695–703.
45. Lipsky BA, Itani K, Norden C, et al. Treating foot infections in diabetic patients: a randomized, multicenter, open-label trial of linezolid versus ampicillin-sulbactam/amoxicillin-clavulanate. Clin Infect Dis 2004;38:17–24.
46. Lipsky BA. New developments in diagnosing and treating diabetic foot infections. Diabetes Metab Res Rev 2008;24(Suppl 1):S66–71.
47. Moran GJ, Krishnadasan A, Gorwitz RJ, et al. Methicillin-resistant *S. aureus* infections among patients in the emergency department. N Engl J Med 2006;355:666–74.
48. Kuck EM, Bouter KP, Hoekstra JB, et al. Tissue concentrations after a single-dose, orally administered ofloxacin in patients with diabetic foot infections. Foot Ankle Int 1998;19:38–40.
49. Raymakers JT, Houben AJ, Heyden JJ, et al. The effect of diabetes and severe ischaemia on the penetration of ceftazidime into tissues of the limb. Diabetic Med 2001;18:229–34.
50. Lipsky BA, Holroyd KJ, Zasloff M. Topical versus systemic antimicrobial therapy for treating mildly infected diabetic foot ulcers: a randomized, controlled, double-blinded, multicenter trial of pexiganan cream. Clin Infect Dis 2008;47(12):1537–45.
51. Baal JG. Surgical treatment of the infected diabetic foot. Clin Infect Dis 2004;39(Suppl 2):S123–8.
52. Tan JS, Friedman NM, Hazelton-Miller C, et al. Can aggressive treatment of diabetic foot infections reduce the need for above-ankle amputation? Clin Infect Dis 1996;23:286–91.
53. Rauwerda JA. Surgical treatment of the infected diabetic foot. Diabetes Metab Res Rev 2004;20(Suppl 1):S41–4.
54. Game F. The advantages and disadvantages of non-surgical management of the diabetic foot. Diabetes Metab Res Rev 2008;24(Suppl 1):S72–5.
55. Lazzarini L, Lipsky BA, Mader JT. Antibiotic treatment of osteomyelitis: what have we learned from 30 years of clinical trials? Int J Infect Dis 2005;9:127–38.

56. Jeffcoate WJ, Lipsky BA. Controversies in diagnosing and managing osteomyelitis of the foot in diabetes. Clin Infect Dis 2004;39(Suppl 2):S115–22.
57. Henke PK, Blackburn SA, Wainess RW, et al. Osteomyelitis of the foot and toe in adults is a surgical disease: conservative management worsens lower extremity salvage. Ann Surg 2005;241:885–92.
58. Senneville E, Lombart A, Beltrand E, et al. Outcome of diabetic foot osteomyelitis treated nonsurgically: a retrospective cohort study. Diabetes Care 2008;31: 637–42.
59. Game FL, Jeffcoate WJ. Primarily nonsurgical management of osteomyelitis of the foot in diabetes. Diabetologia 2008;51:962–7.
60. Eneroth M, Houtum WH. The value of debridement and Vacuum-Assisted Closure (V.A.C.) therapy in diabetic foot ulcers. Diabetes Metab Res Rev 2008;24 (Suppl 1):S76–80.
61. Armstrong D, Lavery L. Negative pressure wound therapy after partial diabetic foot amputation: a multicentre, randomised controlled trial. Lancet 2005;366: 1704–10.
62. Blume PA, Walters J, Payne W, et al. Comparison of negative pressure wound therapy using vacuum-assisted closure with advanced moist wound therapy in the treatment of diabetic foot ulcers: a multicenter randomized controlled trial. Diabetes Care 2008;31:631–6.
63. Roeckl-Wiedmann I, Bennett M, Kranke P. Systematic review of hyperbaric oxygen in the management of chronic wounds. Br J Surg;92:24.
64. Cruciani M, Lipsky BA, Mengoli C, et al. Are granulocyte colony-stimulating factors beneficial in treating diabetic foot infections?: A meta-analysis. Diabetes Care 2005;28:454–60.
65. Eldor R, Raz I, Ben Yehuda A, et al. New and experimental approaches to treatment of diabetic foot ulcers: a comprehensive review of emerging treatment strategies. Diabetic Med 2004;21:1161–73.

Update on Peripheral Arterial Disease and Claudication Rehabilitation

Maya J. Salameh, MD[a,b,]*, Elizabeth V. Ratchford, MD[c,d]

KEYWORDS

- Peripheral arterial disease • Claudication
- Ankle-brachial index • Exercise therapy
- Claudication rehabilitation • Medical management

UPDATE ON PERIPHERAL ARTERIAL DISEASE

Peripheral arterial disease (PAD) is an atherosclerotic syndrome in which the lumen of the arteries in the lower extremities becomes progressively obstructed by plaque. Although technically PAD can also refer to disease in other vascular beds, exclusive of the coronary vessels, in this article the authors refer to PAD as an arterial occlusive disease affecting the lower extremity arteries.

EPIDEMIOLOGY AND RISK FACTORS

Recent epidemiologic projections indicate a prevalence of PAD of 11% to 16% in the population aged 55 years or older, affecting an estimated 27 million persons in Europe and North America alone.[1–3] Moreover, the prevalence of PAD may be as high as 20% to 30% in specific high-risk populations.[4–6] The reported prevalence of PAD depends on the population selected for testing and the methods used for diagnosis.[7] At the start, intermittent claudication questionnaires were used to estimate the prevalence

[a] Division of Cardiology, Department of Medicine, Columbia University College of Physicians and Surgeons, 161 Fort Washington Avenue, Suite 533, New York, NY 10032, USA
[b] Cardiovascular Ultrasound Laboratory, Columbia University Medical Center, 161 Fort Washington Avenue, Suite 533, New York, NY 10032, USA
[c] Division of Cardiology, Department of Medicine, Johns Hopkins University School of Medicine, 600 N. Wolfe Street, Carnegie 568, Baltimore, MD 21287, USA
[d] Department of Medicine, Johns Hopkins Center for Vascular Medicine, 600 N. Wolfe Street, Carnegie 568, Baltimore, MD 21287, USA
* Corresponding author. Division of Cardiology, Department of Medicine, Columbia University College of Physicians and Surgeons, 161 Fort Washington Avenue, Suite 533, New York, NY 10032.
E-mail address: ms3033@columbia.edu (M. Salameh).

Phys Med Rehabil Clin N Am 20 (2009) 627–656
doi:10.1016/j.pmr.2009.06.004
1047-9651/09/$ – see front matter © 2009 Elsevier Inc. All rights reserved.

of PAD in a specific population. Later, a noninvasive test known as the ankle-brachial index (ABI) was developed for a more objective assessment of PAD.[8,9] The ABI is calculated by dividing the ankle systolic pressure by the higher brachial systolic pressure, with an ABI less than 0.9 considered up to 95% sensitive and 99% specific for angiographically confirmed lower extremity arterial disease[10] and a reported positive predictive value of 90%, a negative predictive value of 99%, and an overall accuracy of 98%.[11] One study conducted among 613 individuals living in Southern California used several different techniques to assess the presence of PAD.[12] The study reported that the use of a claudication questionnaire alone significantly underestimated the prevalence of PAD, whereas the use of the ABI combined with pulse wave velocity measurements increased the detection of PAD 2 to 7 times more than claudication symptoms alone. In this study, the prevalence of PAD based on ABI less than 0.9 was 18.8% among those aged 70 years or older, in comparison to a prevalence of 2.5% in those aged 60 years or younger.[12]

Other epidemiologic studies have also described an increase in the prevalence of PAD with increasing age, 1 of the most important risk factors for the development of PAD. For example, the National Health and Nutrition Examination Survey (NHANES), a cross-sectional US survey of 2174 individuals, reported a prevalence of PAD (defined by ABI <0.9) of 14.5% in those aged 70 years or older, compared with a prevalence of 4.3% in the overall population aged 40 years or older.[13] Male gender was previously considered an important risk factor for PAD, but subsequent studies have shown that while men are slightly more affected than women in the younger age groups, the distribution of PAD in the older age groups seems equal between genders.

In epidemiologic studies, race-ethnicity has also emerged as a determining factor for the presence of PAD. NHANES reported that the prevalence of PAD in non-Hispanic blacks was as high as 7.8%, compared with 4.4% in whites.[12] The Multi-Ethnic Study of Atherosclerosis (MESA) also reported a higher prevalence of PAD in blacks compared with whites and Hispanics.[14] Although NHANES and MESA showed a lower prevalence of PAD in Hispanics compared with non-Hispanic whites, Morrissey and colleagues[15] reported that Hispanics present with more advanced stages of disease, demonstrating higher rates of limb-threatening ischemia, failed lower extremity revascularization, and amputations than non-Hispanic whites.

As illustrated in **Fig. 1**, additional risk factors that increase the likelihood of PAD are similar to traditional risk factors for atherosclerosis, including smoking, diabetes mellitus, hypertension, dyslipidemia, chronic kidney disease, hyperhomocysteinemia, and elevated C-reactive protein.[16] Of those, the 2 most strongly associated with PAD are smoking and diabetes. Up to 80% of PAD patients report being current or former smokers.[4] Smoking increases the risk of PAD by 2- to 6-fold,[17] and is twice more likely to cause PAD than coronary artery disease (CAD).[18] Diabetes mellitus, present in up to 20% of patients with PAD, increases the risk of PAD by up to 4-fold;[19] in addition, PAD patients with diabetes are at increased risk for developing lower extremity complications such as major limb amputations.

CLINICAL MANIFESTATIONS OF PAD
Intermittent Claudication and Atypical Leg Symptoms

Intermittent claudication, defined as reproducible pain in the lower limbs during exercise relieved by rest, is the most common manifestation of symptomatic PAD.[7] Claudication most commonly refers to pain in the lower extremity muscle groups, though other symptoms such as fatigue, weakness, or other discomfort may also occur.

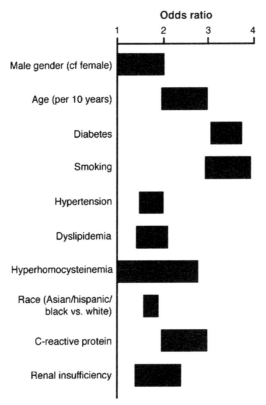

Fig. 1. Risk factors for PAD. The approximate odds ratios for the risk factors for PAD. (*Reprinted from* Norgren L, Hiatt WR, Dormandy JA, et al. on behalf of the TASC-II Working Group. Inter-Society Consensus for the Management of Peripheral Arterial Disease (TASC-II). J Vasc Surg 2007;45 Suppl S:S9A, copyright 2007, Elsevier; with permission.)

Although patients with symptomatic PAD often have sufficient blood flow at rest to avoid limb discomfort, blood flow during exercise is insufficient to meet increased metabolic demands and muscle pain develops. Pain in specific muscle groups is frequently associated with the anatomic site of arterial occlusive disease. For example, pain in the muscles of the buttocks or thighs may represent aortoiliac disease, whereas pain in the calf is most commonly associated with stenosis of the femoral or popliteal arteries.

Several questionnaires have been developed for use in epidemiologic assessments of intermittent claudication. The earliest of these is the Rose Claudication Questionnaire, which has been demonstrated to have high specificity but low sensitivity.[4,5,20,21] Although claudication is considered the main symptom of PAD,[7] it is important to remember that the prevalence of intermittent claudication is low among patients diagnosed with PAD and that several studies have shown that physicians who rely on a history of claudication alone to detect PAD will miss most cases.[5] The Rotterdam Study, which examined 7715 elderly subjects in a population-based study, reported a prevalence of PAD (defined as ABI <0.9) of 19.1%. However, only 1.6% of individuals with PAD reported symptoms of claudication based on the Rose Questionnaire.[4] Newer and more sensitive questionnaires have been developed to determine the presence of lower extremity symptoms, allowing for the assessment of atypical leg pain. For example, the San Diego Questionnaire was developed to categorize patients as having intermittent claudication, atypical leg pain, or no leg pain.[22] This questionnaire was used in the PAD Awareness, Risk and Treatment: New Resources for Survival (PARTNERS) program in which only 8.7% of patients with PAD had a positive Rose Questionnaire.[5] More than half of the patients with PAD exhibited atypical leg symptoms by the San Diego Questionnaire.[5]

Although patients with PAD may have claudication or atypical leg pain, these symptoms are not often brought to the attention of their physicians for a variety of reasons. One study reported that up to one third of patients do not alert a physician to their leg symptoms as they attribute them to musculoskeletal pain, arthritis, or aging.[23] In that same study, patients with objective PAD also demonstrated 1 or more comorbidities such as neuropathy, arthritis, and spinal stenosis. These comorbidities can mask or alter the symptoms of claudication and, as a consequence, physicians may be less likely to consider the diagnosis of PAD in these patients.

Asymptomatic Functional Impairment

Although many patients with PAD may not exhibit symptoms of claudication, evidence suggests that some degree of functional impairment is usually present and that whether or not symptoms develop may depend on the patient's degree of physical activity. The Women's Health and Aging Study examined the lower extremity functioning of 933 women, 328 of whom had PAD as defined by ABI less than 0.9.[24] In the cohort of patients with PAD, 63% reported no leg symptoms with exertion and were therefore classified as asymptomatic; however, after objective testing, these individuals were found to have worse lower extremity functioning than an age-matched cohort.[24] Women who were classified as having asymptomatic PAD were actually found to have slower walking velocities and poorer standing balance scores, and walked fewer blocks per week than women without PAD, after adjustment for other comorbidities.[24] In another cross-sectional study of 460 subjects with PAD and 130 subjects without PAD, McDermott and colleagues[23] reported decreased functional status in subjects with PAD who reported no lower extremity symptoms with exertion. In fact, most subjects with asymptomatic PAD developed symptoms during a 6-minute walk test, suggesting that they were restricting their physical activity in daily life to avoid exertional leg pain.[23] Although a significant number of patients with PAD may be classified as asymptomatic, recent research points to the fact that impaired lower extremity functioning is almost always present in these individuals.

Critical Limb Ischemia

Critical limb ischemia (CLI) is defined by pain in the lower extremities that occurs with rest or evidence of tissue loss in the setting of severely compromised arterial flow. In individuals with CLI, occlusive disease progresses to the point that blood flow at rest becomes insufficient for tissue viability, and chronic rest pain, ulcers, or gangrene can develop. The natural history of CLI is not well defined as most of these patients now receive early invasive treatment. However, if untreated, the expected outcome would be major limb amputation within 6 months.[17] Patients with CLI usually present with foot pain at rest that may worsen in the supine position and may improve when the limb is placed in a dependent position. Although fewer than 5% to 10% of patients with PAD have CLI, patients with diabetes are particularly prone to developing this syndrome, which is associated with a substantial risk of limb loss.[25] Acute limb ischemia (ALI) occurs due to a sudden deterioration in limb perfusion and may be a form of CLI but is more commonly related to an acute event such as embolism or local thrombosis. Patients with ALI often present with the 5 "Ps" of pain, pallor, paresthesias, pulselessness, and poikilothermia and commonly report no prior history of claudication. ALI, which is associated with a high mortality and significant risk of limb loss,[7] should be treated emergently, usually with a combination of anticoagulation therapy, thrombolysis, and open surgical repair.

NATURAL HISTORY OF PAD
Cardiovascular Outcomes

Given the coexistence of coronary and cerebrovascular disease in patients with PAD, as well as a well-described association between ABI and cardiovascular morbidity and mortality, patients with PAD are considered at significantly increased risk for myocardial infarction, stroke, and vascular death over a 5-year period in comparison to age-matched cohorts. The overall 5-year mortality for PAD patients is approximately 15% to 30%, with more than 75% attributable to cardiovascular causes.[17]

PAD as a marker for disease in other vascular beds
Prior studies have demonstrated that patients with symptomatic atherosclerotic disease in 1 vascular bed are at risk for polyvascular disease. For example, 26% of patients analyzed as part of the Clopidogrel versus Aspirin in Patients at Risk of Ischemic Events (CAPRIE) trial had symptomatic disease in at least 2 vascular beds.[26] The Swiss Atherothrombosis Survey revealed that 52% of symptomatic PAD patients reported a concurrent history of stroke/transient ischemic attack (TIA) or CAD and that 23% of patients with a history of stroke/TIA or CAD were found to have previously undiagnosed, asymptomatic PAD.[27] The recent Reduction of Atherothrombosis for Continued Health (REACH) international registry which includes 63,000 patients from 43 countries has demonstrated that 63% of approximately 7000 patients with PAD have concomitant symptomatic cerebrovascular or coronary disease.[28]

The ABI and vascular events
The Framingham Heart Study initially described the association between intermittent claudication and both coronary heart disease and stroke and reported a 2-fold age-adjusted increased risk of death in men and women with claudication.[29] The presence of PAD as defined by an ABI less than 0.9 has been associated with a 6-fold increased risk of cardiovascular death at 10 years[30] and a 2- to 3-fold increased risk of ischemic stroke[31] when compared with the general population. Although an ABI between 0.9 and 1.3 has been traditionally considered normal,[5] the MESA has reported excess coronary and carotid atherosclerosis in subjects with low-normal ABIs (0.9–1.1) and high ABIs (>1.3), suggesting that even subjects with borderline or low-normal ABIs may be at increased risk for cardiovascular events.[14] Medial calcification, or incompressible arteries, common in the elderly and in patients with long-standing diabetes or chronic kidney disease, may also be associated with higher cardiovascular risk. For example, the Strong Heart Study reported an increased risk of all-cause and cardiovascular mortality for subjects with a low ABI (<0.9), borderline ABI (0.9–1.0), and high ABI (>1.4).[32]

Limb Outcomes

For PAD patients presenting with CLI, the prognosis of the limb is poor in the absence of timely revascularization. However, in patients initially presenting with intermittent claudication or atypical leg pain, limb symptoms typically stabilize over time, with only 10% to 20% of patients experiencing worsening claudication and fewer than 2% progressing to CLI.[17] For patients with PAD who are initially asymptomatic, a degree of functional decline over time has been described. One study revealed that PAD patients who were asymptomatic at baseline had significantly greater decline in walking performance at 2 years than those without PAD.[33]

NONINVASIVE DIAGNOSIS OF PAD
History and Physical Examination

The diagnosis of PAD should begin with a thorough history. PAD should be considered in patients presenting with symptoms suggestive of claudication or in patients with multiple risk factors for PAD and atypical leg pain. The differential diagnosis of exertional leg pain also includes spinal stenosis, osteoarthritis, peripheral neuropathy, and venous claudication.

The physical examination should be conducted with the patient in a gown with shoes and socks off, with a focus on skin changes, pulses, and the presence or absence of ulcers. Skin findings common in PAD include abnormal color (red or dusky purple) or pallor, hair loss on legs and toes, cool skin, and atrophic nail changes.[34] In the setting of severe arterial insufficiency, ulcers may be present either on the toes or on the lateral malleolus. Arterial ulcers are usually painful (unless the patient has a concomitant peripheral neuropathy) and may be associated with a surrounding cellulitis or gangrene. Assessment of the femoral, popliteal, posterior tibial, and dorsalis pedis pulses should also be part of the physical examination. The femoral pulse can be palpated inferior to the inguinal ligament. The absence of a femoral pulse may indicate a stenosis or occlusion of the distal aorta or iliac artery. The popliteal pulse is felt in the popliteal fossa behind the knee. A prominent popliteal pulse may be suggestive of a popliteal artery aneurysm, while a diminished or absent pulse may indicate more proximal stenosis. The posterior tibial artery is found posterior to the medial malleolus and the dorsalis pedis artery on the dorsum of the foot.

It is important to remember that a pulse examination alone is not sufficient to establish the diagnosis of PAD. Criqui and colleagues[21] reported that an abnormal dorsalis pedis artery pulse was 50% sensitive and 73% specific for the detection of PAD, whereas an abnormal posterior tibial artery pulse demonstrated a sensitivity of 71% and a specificity of 91%. A handheld Doppler device, along with acoustic gel, can be used to assess the arterial signal. A normal arterial signal contains 3 components and is described as triphasic. In the presence of disease, the arterial signal is altered and may only have 2 components (biphasic) or 1 component (monophasic). In cases of severe disease or occlusion, the arterial signal may be absent. Other physical findings that may be suggestive of PAD include the presence of a bruit by auscultation of the iliac, femoral, or popliteal arteries. One study which reviewed the accuracy of the clinical examination for PAD reported that the presence of a femoral bruit significantly increases the likelihood of PAD; however, its absence does not affect the probability that PAD is present.[34]

ABI

The ABI is considered the most effective PAD screening test.[8,9] The ABI is measured after the patient has been lying supine for 5 to 10 minutes. The systolic pressure is measured at the bilateral brachial, dorsalis pedis, and posterior tibial arteries using appropriately sized (10–12 cm) sphygmomanometer cuffs and a handheld 5- or 10-MHz Doppler probe with acoustic gel (**Fig. 2**). Typically, the ABI for each leg is calculated by dividing the higher of the 2 ankle pressures in that leg by the higher of the 2 brachial pressures. The lower of the left and right ABI values is reported as the ABI.[16] An ABI less than 0.9 is diagnostic of PAD and also gives information regarding the severity of disease; specifically, an ABI of 0.7 to 0.89 is considered mild, an ABI of

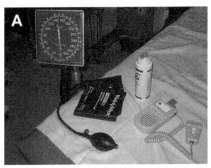
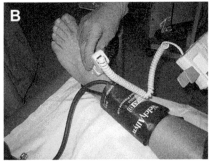
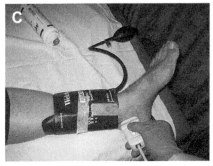

Fig. 2. How to measure the ABI. (*A*) Appropriately sized (10–12 cm) sphygmomanometer cuff, a handheld 5- or 10-MHz. Doppler probe, and acoustic gel are needed to measure the ABI. (*B*) Proper placement of Doppler probe for measurement of the dorsalis pedis pressure. (*C*) Proper placement of Doppler probe for measurement of the posterior tibial pressure.

0.4 to 0.69 is moderate, and an ABI less than 0.4 is severe. The range for a normal ABI is 0.9 to 1.3, though the range from 0.9 to 1.0 is considered borderline or indeterminate (**Fig. 3**).

The ABI has some significant limitations. In some patients, such as the elderly and those with diabetes or chronic kidney disease, calcified or noncompressible vessels can lead to falsely elevated ankle pressures, which may result in an artificially "normal" ABI or a high ABI (>1.3). In certain cases, medial calcification may cause difficulty in abolishing the systolic pressure signal despite inflating the cuff to pressures more than 250 mmHg.[16] Another major limitation of the ABI is that it may seem normal at rest in patients with aortoiliac disease, usually when collaterals are present. The ABI only becomes abnormal with exercise when areas of stenosis or occlusion become hemodynamically significant. Thus, it is important not to exclude the diagnosis of PAD when the resting ABI is normal, particularly if symptoms suggestive of claudication are present. In these instances, the patient may be asked to exercise (usually on a treadmill at 1.5–2 mph at a 12% grade) until the claudication symptoms are reproduced, for a maximum of 5 minutes. The ankle pressure is measured again following exercise, with a 15% to 20% subsequent drop in the ABI considered diagnostic of PAD.[16]

Noninvasive Physiologic Testing

Noninvasive physiologic testing, when added to the ABI, can provide additional key information, including determination of the location and severity of PAD. The

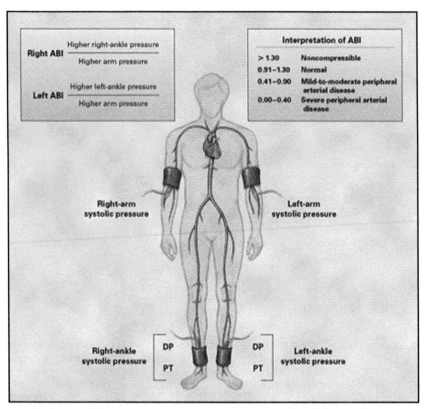

Fig. 3. Calculation of the ABI. The systolic pressure is measured at the bilateral brachial, dorsalis pedis, and posterior tibial arteries. The ABI for each leg is calculated by dividing the higher of the 2 ankle pressures in that leg by the higher of the 2 brachial pressures. An ABI less than 0.9 is diagnostic of PAD and also gives information regarding the severity of disease; specifically, an ABI between 0.7 and 0.89 is considered mild, an ABI between 0.4 and 0.69 is moderate, and an ABI less than 0.4 is severe. In some patients, calcified or noncompressible vessels can lead to falsely elevated ankle pressures, which may result in an artificially "normal" ABI or a high ABI (>1.3). (*Reprinted from* Hiatt WR. Drug therapy: medical treatment of peripheral arterial disease and claudication. N Engl J Med 2001;344:1610, copyright 2001, Massachusetts Medical Society, all rights reserved; with permission.)

components of physiologic testing include segmental limb pressures and pulse volume recordings (PVRs). Continuous wave Doppler tracings are also an alternative to PVRs. Segmental limb systolic pressures are measured using sphygmomanometer cuffs at the thigh, calf, and ankle levels. PVRs are obtained using plethysmography, a technique whereby air is inflated into each cuff up to a pressure of 65 mmHg. The transient volume change beneath the cuff is then translated into a pulsatile waveform. PVRs can provide valuable information about the presence of PAD, especially in cases in which the ABI may be artificially normal or elevated due to calcified vessels. An example of the noninvasive physiologic testing method is shown in **Fig. 4**. **Fig. 5** contains examples of normal and abnormal physiologic test results.

Noninvasive physiologic testing provides adequate information regarding the presence or absence of PAD, its severity, which segments are likely involved; however,

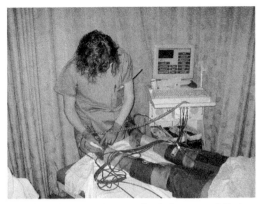

Fig. 4. The noninvasive physiologic testing method. Segmental limb systolic pressures are measured using sphygmomanometer cuffs at the thigh, calf, and ankle levels. PVRs are obtained using plethysmography, a technique whereby air is inflated into each cuff up to a pressure of 65 mmHg and the transient volume change beneath the cuff is translated into a pulsatile waveform.

further imaging is indicated when more specific information about the degree and exact location of PAD is needed, often in the case of planning before a procedure. The goal of imaging in PAD is to determine the location of disease (inflow vs outflow), whether stenoses or occlusions are confined to discrete or long segments, and severity of disease. Imaging may also help determine whether the patient is a better candidate for endovascular or surgical revascularization and may help in procedural planning. If endovascular revascularization is a consideration, further imaging can also help to provide information about the likelihood of long-term patency to assist the patient and the physician in the decision making process.

Arterial Duplex

Arterial duplex can be used as an adjunct to physiologic testing for assessing the presence and location of lower extremity PAD. Duplex testing is more costly and can be time-consuming. The technique is also dependent on the proficiency of the operator.[35] Therefore this method is most often used to obtain focused information about the level and severity of arterial stenoses or occlusions, the patency of bypass grafts or stents, and the presence of pseudoaneurysms or arteriovenous fistulas. In the presence of stenosis, Doppler evaluation demonstrates elevated flow velocities within the stenotic arterial segment. Generally, at least a doubling of the velocity at the site of stenosis in comparison to a proximal normal segment indicates hemodynamically significant stenosis (**Fig. 6**).

CTA and MRA

Computed tomography angiography (CTA) and magnetic resonance angiography (MRA) are considered highly sensitive and specific in the evaluation of PAD. CTA is inexpensive and quick, offering excellent visualization of inflow disease and surgical bypasses. However, CTA requires radiation exposure, although less than that required for catheter-based angiography.[36] MRA, which is comparable to CTA in terms of inflow and surgical bypass visualization, is particularly useful for visualization of tibial vessels[37] and also does not result in ionizing radiation exposure. MRA, however, is more costly than CTA and not as readily available; MRA is also contraindicated in patients with pacemakers or defibrillators. In addition, the risk of nephrogenic systemic fibrosis has been described in patients with Stages 4 or 5 chronic kidney disease who are exposed to gadolinium.[38] Other limitations of MRA include difficulty with calcium visualization and inadequate assessment of peripheral stents due to

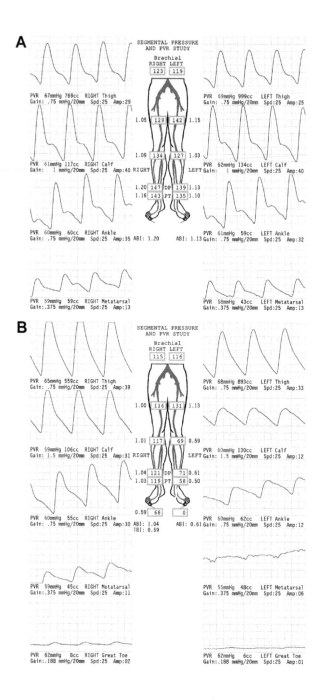

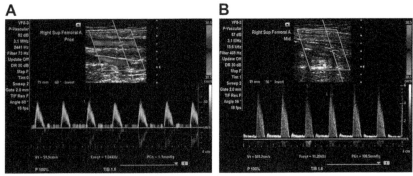

Fig. 6. Measurement of superficial femoral artery stenosis using arterial duplex. (*A*) Arterial duplex image and spectral Doppler waveform analysis of the proximal superficial femoral artery. The velocity obtained within that segment is within normal limits at 51.9 cm/s (normal < 200 cm/s). (*B*) Arterial duplex image and spectral Doppler waveform analysis of the mid superficial femoral artery at the level of stenosis in the same patient. An elevated velocity of 501.2 cm/s (normal < 200 cm/s) is obtained. The ratio of the velocity at the level of stenosis to the velocity in the normal proximal segment is 9.6; a ratio ≥2 is consistent with ≥50% stenosis. This velocity indicates significant stenosis at the level of the mid superficial femoral artery.

artifact. For peripheral stent evaluation, CTA or arterial duplex is the preferred imaging modality.

Contrast Arteriography

Digital substraction arteriography (DSA) is often considered the gold standard for arterial imaging, with improved spatial resolution over CTA or MRA.[39] DSA also offers the opportunity for endovascular revascularization during the diagnostic procedure. However, contrast toxicity, cost, and complications associated with arterial puncture make DSA difficult to use routinely as a diagnostic method for lower extremity PAD.

MEDICAL MANAGEMENT OF PAD

The management of PAD should follow a 3-pronged approach: (1) identification and treatment of systemic atherosclerosis, (2) improvement of functional status, and (3) preservation of the limb. These therapeutic goals must be addressed simultaneously,

---

Fig. 5. Noninvasive physiologic testing results. (*A*) Example of a normal noninvasive physiologic test. Segmental pressures are obtained at the brachial, thigh, calf, and ankle levels. Pressures are compared level to level and side to side. A drop of 20 mmHg or more between segments is considered significant and helps to localize the disease. In this case, no significant pressure drops are noted and ABIs are in the normal range. PVRs are normal, demonstrating a sharp upstroke, a distinct peak, and a dicrotic notch during diastole. (*B*) Example of an abnormal noninvasive physiologic test. The PVR tracings seem moderately abnormal at the left calf and ankle with loss of amplitude and a rounded waveform. The PVR tracing at the left metatarsal is severely abnormal. A large drop in pressure is noted between the left thigh and calf, indicating femoral-popliteal disease. The ABI on the left is 0.61 which is in the moderately abnormal range. On the right, the PVR tracings seem within normal limits, with a preserved upstroke, a distinct peak, and a dicrotic notch. Accordingly, the ABI on the right is in the normal range.

as each has a significant impact on the long-term outcomes of patients with PAD, in terms of mortality benefit and improved quality of life (**Box 1**).

Treatment of Systemic Atherosclerosis for Cardiovascular Risk Reduction

Given the systemic nature of atherosclerosis, patients with PAD are at high risk for developing cardiovascular events such as myocardial infarction and stroke. Aggressive cardiovascular risk reduction should be a central component of the medical management of PAD.

Antiplatelet agents

Treatment with antiplatelet agents is recommended to reduce the risk of recurrent vascular events (myocardial infarction, ischemic stroke, or vascular death) in patients with lower extremity PAD.[17] The data supporting this recommendation are mainly derived from the Antiplatelet Trialists' Collaboration, a meta-analysis of 287 studies of antiplatelet agents.[40] The meta-analysis included 135,000 patients who had clinical cardiovascular disease, including 9214 patients with PAD. In the PAD subgroup treated with antiplatelet therapy, there was a 22% odds reduction for adverse cardiovascular events, defined as myocardial infarction, stroke, or vascular death.[40] The

---

Box 1
Management of PAD

Treatment of systemic atherosclerosis for cardiovascular risk reduction

    Antiplatelet agents

    Lipid-modifying agents such as 3-hydroxy-3-methylglutaryl coenzyme A (HMG CoA) reductase inhibitors to target low density lipoprotein cholesterol (LDL-C) less than 100 mg/dL (can consider target LDL-C<70 mg/dL in selected cases)

    Treatment of blood pressure to achieve a target less than 140/90 or less than 130/80 mmHg if concomitant diabetes or chronic kidney disease

    Angiotensin-converting enzyme (ACE) inhibitors (or angiotensin receptor blockers)

    Treatment of diabetes to achieve hemoglobin A1C goal of less than 7.0%

    Smoking cessation

Improvement of functional status and quality of life

    Cilostazol

    Exercise training, preferably supervised

    Diet and weight loss

    Endovascular revascularization in selected cases

    Surgical revascularization in selected cases

Preservation of the limb

    Meticulous foot care

    Treatment of diabetes to achieve hemoglobin A1C goal of less than 7.0%

    Smoking cessation

    Endovascular revascularization

    Surgical revascularization

most common antiplatelet therapy used in these trials was aspirin. In comparing the efficacy of different doses of aspirin, the meta-analysis reported comparable proportional reductions in vascular events between 75 to 150 mg daily and 160 to 325 mg daily ranges. There was a significantly lower reduction in risk in those patients treated with less than 75 mg of aspirin daily.[40] Current guidelines support the use of aspirin in daily doses of 75 to 325 mg to reduce the risk of cardiovascular events in patients with lower extremity PAD.[17]

Clopidogrel, a thienopyridine drug, has been evaluated in the CAPRIE trial.[26] This trial randomized approximately 19,000 patients with recent myocardial infarction, recent ischemic stroke, or moderately severe symptomatic PAD to 75 mg of clopidogrel daily versus 325 mg of aspirin daily. In the PAD subgroup, which consisted of 6452 patients with claudication and an ABI less than 0.85 or prior lower extremity bypass surgery, angioplasty, or amputation, those treated with clopidogrel had a 23.8% relative risk reduction for vascular events compared with those treated with aspirin.[26] Based on the results of the CAPRIE trial subgroup analysis, current guidelines support clopidogrel 75 mg daily as an "effective alternative antiplatelet therapy to aspirin" in the prevention of vascular events in patients with lower extremity PAD.[17] There is no current evidence to support the use of combination therapy with aspirin and clopidogrel for cardiovascular risk reduction in patients with lower extremity PAD.

Smoking cessation

Cigarette smoking is considered an important risk factor for the development of PAD, with a 3- to 6-fold increased risk of intermittent claudication in smokers versus nonsmokers.[39] In addition, 1 study revealed that smokers with PAD developed claudication more quickly while walking than nonsmokers with PAD, and their leg symptoms took longer to subside.[41] Although there have been no randomized controlled trials comparing outcomes in smokers versus nonsmokers with PAD, it has been demonstrated that smoking cessation in patients with PAD decreases the risk of future cardiovascular events and reduces progression to lower extremity CLI.[25] In PAD patients who continue to smoke, the 10-year mortality has been reported to be as high as 40% to 50%, with most deaths due to stroke or myocardial infarction.[39]

The approach to smoking cessation includes education, counseling, and the use of pharmacologic therapy. Several pharmacologic agents have been approved for use in smoking cessation. Nicotine replacement therapy (NRT) is a good first-line approach, given that the chemical addiction to nicotine is believed to drive patients to keep smoking. Nicotine replacement, which is considered safe in patients with vascular disease, can be achieved through several different modalities, including gum, spray, inhaler, or patch.[39] Another pharmacologic agent is bupropion hydrochloride (Zyban), which has been shown to increase smoking cessation rates over placebo, from 12% in patients using placebo to 23% in those using bupropion.[42]

Another agent, varenicline, has recently become available to aid in smoking cessation. Varenicline is a partial agonist of nicotinic acetylcholine receptors and has been shown in 2 randomized trials to be superior to bupropion and placebo in continuous abstinence rates at 12 and 24 weeks.[43,44] However, concerns have arisen regarding the safety of varenicline, with a variety of reported adverse effects including falls, syncope, and vision disturbances.[45] More importantly, the US Food and Drug Administration (FDA) recently advised health care providers that suicidal thoughts and aggressive behavior have also been reported in patients taking varenicline.[45] Thus, varenicline must be used cautiously in patients who qualify for treatment, with increased vigilance on the part of physicians for the development of serious adverse effects. NRT can be prescribed in conjunction with bupropion but is not recommended with varenicline due to the mechanism of action.

Diabetes

Patients with diabetes mellitus have a 2- to 4-fold increased risk for developing PAD in comparison to patients without diabetes.[17,19] One study revealed that the prevalence of PAD in diabetic patients was as high as 22.4% compared with 12.5% in patients without diabetes.[46] This same study also demonstrated a high prevalence of PAD in patients with impaired glucose tolerance, up to 19.9% compared with 12.5% in patients with normal glucose tolerance.[46] Patients with diabetes are also at increased risk for developing intermittent claudication and are more likely to develop infrapopliteal occlusive disease in comparison to nondiabetic subjects.[47] Tight glycemic control has not been shown to reduce the incidence of intermittent claudication or rest pain. However, the UK Prospective Diabetes Study revealed that tight control of glucose decreases microvascular complications and may also decrease the risk of myocardial infarction.[48] In addition, meticulous foot care is critical in PAD patients with diabetes, given their higher risk of developing limb ischemia and ulcerations.

Dyslipidemia

The NHANES study demonstrated that dyslipidemia is strongly associated with lower extremity PAD.[13] Another study reported that the odds of developing PAD increase by approximately 10% for every 10 mg/dL increase in total cholesterol.[49] The Heart Protection Study, which included 20,536 patients at high risk for cardiovascular events, including 6748 patients with PAD, randomized subjects to treatment with simvastatin (40 mg) versus placebo.[50] Within the PAD subgroup, there was a 25% relative risk reduction in vascular events at 5 years in subjects treated with simvastatin, including in patients with normal LDL levels at baseline.[50] The Scandinavian Simvastatin Survival Study demonstrated that subjects in the PAD subgroup treated with simvastatin had a lower likelihood of new or worsening claudication than those treated with placebo.[51] Given that dylipidemia is considered a risk factor for developing PAD, and that treatment of dyslipidemia results in a reduction in major cardiovascular events in PAD patients, the National Cholesterol Education Program Adult Treatment Panel III has recommended similar lipid treatment strategies for patients with PAD as for those with CAD.[52] As a result, current guidelines support the use of HMG CoA reductase inhibitor (statin) medications in patients with PAD with a goal LDL of less than 100 mg/dL. A target LDL of less than 70 mg/dL may be considered in PAD patients with multiple major risk factors including diabetes, poorly controlled risk factors such as current cigarette smoking, or multiple risk factors of the metabolic syndrome.[17,52]

Hypertension

Hypertension is considered an independent risk factor for PAD.[3,29] No data are available to confirm that treatment of hypertension reduces progression of lower extremity PAD or the incidence of intermittent claudication, though prior evidence supports treatment of hypertension to improve cardiovascular outcomes. For example, the Appropriate Blood Pressure Control in Diabetes trial included 950 patients with diabetes, 53 of whom had PAD defined by ABI less than 0.9. Subjects were randomized to moderate or intensive blood pressure treatment and followed for 5 years. The cardiovascular event rate in PAD patients receiving intensive blood pressure treatment was 13.6% compared with an event rate of 38.7% in those receiving moderate treatment; these results suggest that intensive blood pressure control has the potential of reducing cardiovascular events in PAD patients with diabetes.[53] According to current guidelines, blood pressure should be managed to a goal of less than 140 mmHg systolic over 90 mmHg diastolic in all patients with PAD, with a further blood pressure goal of less than 130 mmHg systolic over 80 mmHg diastolic in patients who have concomitant diabetes mellitus or chronic kidney disease.[17] Some concern was reported regarding the use of β-adrenergic antagonist drugs (β-blockers) for the treatment of hypertension in PAD patients based on previous case reports that β-blockers reduced lower extremity blood flow and led to an increase in claudication symptoms.[25] However, subsequent studies have not reported any adverse events with the use of β-blockers; a meta-analysis of these studies concluded that β-blockers do not affect walking ability in patients with PAD.[54]

Evidence suggests that ACE inhibitors may reduce the risk of cardiovascular events in patients with PAD beyond that expected from blood pressure control alone. The Heart Outcomes Prevention Evaluation (HOPE) study randomized 9257 high-risk patients to treatment with ramipril (an ACE inhibitor) versus placebo. Treatment with ramipril reduced the 5-year event rate (a composite of myocardial infarction, stroke, or vascular death) from 17.7% in the placebo group to 14.4% in the ramipril group. The benefit of ACE inhibition was also noted in the PAD subgroup, which included 4051 patients with PAD defined by ABI less than 0.9.[55] The more recent Ongoing Telmisartan Alone and in combination with Ramipril Global Endpoint trial (ON TARGET) trial demonstrated that telimsartan, an angiotensin II receptor blocker, was equivalent to ramipril in prevention of cardiovascular events, including in the subgroup of patients with PAD.[56] Current guidelines support the use of ACE inhibitors or angiotensin receptor blockers to reduce the risk of cardiovascular events in patients with lower extremity PAD.[17]

Improvement of Functional Status and Quality of Life

Patients with intermittent claudication have reduced functional capacity and impaired exercise tolerance, often leading to difficulty in performing activities of daily living.[25] Symptoms of claudication can range from mildly disabling to severely lifestyle-limiting, resulting in decreased quality of life. Effective therapy for intermittent claudication is essential to ensure improvement in the functional status of patients with lower extremity PAD, thereby directly enhancing their quality of life. Therapy for claudication includes supervised exercise training, pharmacologic therapy, and lifestyle modification. Supervised exercise training is the most important nonpharmacologic therapy for claudication and has been proven effective in improving pain-free and maximal walking distance in patients with PAD.[57] Supervised exercise therapy is discussed in detail separately in this article.

Pharmacologic therapy: cilostazol

The main pharmacologic agent currently used in the treatment of claudication in patients with PAD is cilostazol, which received FDA approval in 1999. Cilostazol is a phosphodiesterase type 3 inhibitor which increases intracellular cyclic AMP concentrations.[25] Cilostazol also inhibits vascular smooth muscle cell proliferation and platelet aggregation and causes vasodilation.[25] However, neither platelet aggregation nor vasodilation is supported as the mechanism by which cilostazol improves claudication. Five prospective randomized controlled trials have been published to date examining the efficacy of cilostazol over placebo in improving claudication symptoms. The trials have revealed that cilostazol increases pain-free and maximal walking distance in PAD patients by 40% to 60% in comparison to placebo.[58–62] A meta-analysis of these trials concluded that in addition to improving walking distance, cilostazol also improves health-related quality of life.[63] The main side effects reported with cilostazol include headache, diarrhea, dizziness, and palpitations.[25] Importantly, cilostazol is contraindicated in heart failure due to the previously observed increased mortality in long-term administration of oral phosphodiesterase type 3 inhibitors such as milrinone in patients with heart failure.[64] A black box warning not to administer cilostazol to claudicants who also have heart failure of any severity is currently in effect.[25]

Pharmacologic therapy: pentoxifylline

Pentoxifylline is a methylxanthine derivative that improves red cell deformability, has mild antiplatelet effects, and lowers plasma fibrinogen.[7] Pentoxifylline was first approved in 1984 for the treatment of claudication based on earlier data that showed a modest improvement in maximal treadmill walking distance in patients treated with pentoxifylline versus placebo.[65] Meta-analyses of the pentoxifylline trials revealed a small but marginal increase in walking distance with the use of pentoxifylline over placebo.[66,67] A more recent study aimed at studying the efficacy of cilostazol versus pentoxifylline and placebo revealed that while cilostazol improved pain-free and maximal walking distance, pentoxifylline was no more effective than placebo in improving either pain-free or maximal walking distance.[62] Therefore, based on available evidence, current guidelines suggest that although pentoxifylline may be considered in the treatment of claudication, it is unlikely to be of significant clinical benefit and its widespread use is therefore not recommended.[17]

Pharmacologic therapy: other agents

Alternative pharmacologic agents and nutritional supplements have been studied in the treatment of claudication. Prostaglandins, which include prostaglandin E1 and oral analogs such as beraprost, have vasodilator properties and inhibit platelet aggregation.[17] Although 1 randomized trial demonstrated that beraprost improved walking distance in patients with claudication,[68] a more recent larger randomized trial found no benefit.[69] Furthermore, beraprost was associated with significant side effects including flushing, headaches, and gastrointestinal effects. Given that available evidence has failed to show the effectiveness of prostaglandins in the treatment of claudication, it is unlikely that this class of drugs will be approved for this indication in the future.[17] Angiogenic growth factors such as vascular endothelial growth factor have also been studied in the treatment of claudication, mainly because they have been shown to increase extremity blood flow and collateral formation in experimental models.[17,70] However, further studies are needed to determine the efficacy of angiogenic growth factors in the treatment of claudication. Nutritional supplements such as L-arginine and gingko biloba have been studied but their efficacy in improving walking distance in patients with claudication is not well established. Vitamin E, which has also been previously studied, is not currently recommended as an effective therapy for claudication.[17]

Revascularization for claudication

Current guidelines support the use of revascularization, whether endovascular or surgical, in selected cases only. Specifically, invasive revascularization for claudication should only be considered once the following factors have been taken into account: (1) response to at least 3 months of exercise or pharmacologic therapies for claudication has been inadequate; (2) a lifestyle-limiting disability due to claudication is present, preventing the patient from performing activities of daily living; (3) the vascular anatomy has been evaluated in terms of suitability for intervention, with a favorable risk to benefit ratio, such as in the case focal aortoiliac disease; and (4) the presence of other comorbid conditions that would otherwise limit the patient's activity have been considered and evaluated before considering lower extremity revascularization.[17] Patient preference also plays a significant role in the decision to proceed with interventional therapy for claudication. Patients should be referred early to a vascular specialist for evaluation and management and to determine if invasive revascularization is indicated.

Once patients have been appropriately selected for revascularization, further imaging with CTA, MRA, or contrast angiography may then be obtained to determine whether the arterial anatomy is more suitable for endovascular versus surgical revascularization. Endovascular revascularization is now used more frequently in the treatment of claudication due to rapid advancements in endovascular techniques, which include angioplasty with balloon dilation, atherectomy, and stenting.[17] Long-term patency seems best in the endovascular treatment of iliac lesions, as compared with more distal lesions, which have lower patency rates over time; patency rates also decrease in the setting of long-segment occlusions, multiple tandem lesions, and poor run-off.[17] Current guidelines recommend endovascular treatment as the preferred revascularization technique for short segment (3 cm or less) single lesions in the iliac or femoropopliteal segments.[17] Surgical revascularization for claudication may also be considered, though it is not performed frequently for this indication in part due to the high cardiovascular risk for surgery in patients with PAD.

Lifestyle modification

Prior studies have shown that PAD patients with impaired lower extremity function demonstrate reduced physical activity levels in comparison to patients with normal lower extremity function, possibly contributing to subsequent disability.[71] Given that patients with intermittent claudication are at the low end of the physical activity spectrum, they may be at increased risk for being overweight or obese. The result of this can lead to the development of the metabolic syndrome, a condition characterized by abdominal obesity, high triglyceride and low high density lipoprotein levels, hypertension, and glucose intolerance.[72] It is particularly important to consider the possible negative consequences that the metabolic syndrome may have on peripheral circulation and ambulation in a population of patients already exhibiting significant limitations on physical functioning.

The metabolic syndrome can exacerbate the ambulatory dysfunction of PAD patients with intermittent claudication, leading to shorter walking distances and poorer health-related quality of life. One study of 423 patients with PAD and stable intermittent claudication revealed that PAD patients with the metabolic syndrome demonstrated shorter initial and absolute claudication distances compared with those PAD patients without the metabolic syndrome.[73] Furthermore, patients with the metabolic syndrome exhibited shorter Walking Impairment Questionnaire (WIQ) distances, lower self-perceived health, and a lower health-related quality of life.[73] Further studies are needed to test interventions designed to treat the risk factors of the metabolic syndrome, particularly insulin sensitivity, to improve physical functioning and long-term prognosis in PAD patients. The Diabetes Prevention Program[74] revealed that exercise and modest weight loss can significantly impact insulin sensitivity and prevent progression to diabetes. There was a 58% reduction in the risk of developing diabetes in patients randomized to lifestyle changes with diet and exercise in comparison to the usual care group.[74] It is reasonable to consider that in addition to preventing the development of diabetes, lifestyle modifications such as changes in diet, increase in daily exercise, and weight loss may also help in improving health-related quality of life in patients with lower extremity PAD, particularly those who are overweight and obese and at risk for developing the metabolic syndrome.

Preservation of the Limb

Meticulous foot care

A key strategy for limb preservation in patients with PAD is prevention of skin break-down which can ultimately lead to ulceration and amputation. Prevention begins with meticulous foot care. Patients with PAD and concomitant diabetes should be evaluated regularly by a podiatry specialist. Patients should also be educated about performing daily foot inspections and using moisturizing creams regularly to prevent dryness. In addition, appropriate footwear should be used to prevent pressure-induced skin breakdown and ulceration.[17]

Invasive therapies for CLI

CLI occurs when blood flow at rest is insufficient for tissue viability. Physical signs of tissue ischemia, such as dependent rubor and elevation pallor, calf atrophy, ischemic ulcers, or gangrene, should lead to rapid evaluation and consideration for lower extremity revascularization for limb salvage. It is estimated that up to 50% of patients with CLI will require revascularization for limb salvage and in those with disease that is not easily treatable invasively, up to 40% will require a major limb amputation within 6 months of presentation.[17] Endovascular and surgical interventions are used in limb salvage, and selection of the specific revascularization strategy may depend in part on the vascular anatomy, the presence of inflow or outflow disease, and patient comorbidities.

UPDATE ON CLAUDICATION REHABILITATION

After the diagnosis of PAD is made, exercise training plays a critical role as a primary treatment of claudication with the goals of improving quality of life and functional capacity. The concept of exercise for treating claudication dates back to a German article published by Erb in 1898.[75] The first randomized controlled trial was published in 1966; a marked improvement in walking ability was seen in PAD patients assigned to daily exercise.[76] According to the American College of Cardiology (ACC)/American Heart Association (AHA) Practice Guidelines for the management of PAD, supervised exercise training is rated as Class I, Level of Evidence A for the initial treatment of claudication.[17] As per these guidelines, the program should be at least 30 to 45 minutes 3 times weekly for at least 12 weeks.[17]

Numerous prospective studies have demonstrated the benefits of exercise training for improving claudication symptoms.[57,77,78] Studies differ in terms of the magnitude of the reported response to exercise which is likely explained by the variability in the exercise intervention itself (duration, frequency, and intensity) as well as in the outcome measures.[79] In a meta-analysis of 21 nonrandomized and randomized studies, Gardner and Poehlman confirmed that exercise training improves claudication symptoms; they found a 179% increase in pain-free walking distance (+225.3 m) and a 122% increase in maximum walking distance (+397.5 m).[57] A Cochrane review of 22 randomized controlled trials for claudication also reported significant improvements, with mean increases in maximum walking time (+5.12 minutes), pain-free walking distance (+82.2 m) and maximum walking distance (+113.20 m).[78]

Supervised exercise training is generally accepted as superior to unsupervised training.[80] A Cochrane review looked at 8 small trials including a total of 319 subjects and found a significant improvement in maximum treadmill walking distance in supervised programs compared with unsupervised programs, with a difference of approximately 150 m.[80]

Only a small number of studies have compared the effectiveness of exercise versus revascularization. For example, in a prospective randomized trial comparing supervised exercise to angioplasty published in 1990, Creasy and colleagues[81] found that mean maximum walking distances progressively increased in the supervised exercise group at 6, 9, and 12 months but did not increase in the angioplasty group even though angioplasty improved the ABIs. A subsequent article from the same study reported that after a median follow-up of 70 months, the functional outcome was the same between the exercise group and the angioplasty group.[82] In the Edinburgh study published in 1997, 62 patients were randomized to angioplasty versus medical treatment.[83] At 2 years, no differences were seen between the 2 groups in terms of treadmill walking distances or quality of life; the medical group was not in a supervised program but was simply given "exercise advice" to walk at home.

The relative benefit of supervised exercise versus endovascular revascularization is not known, particularly in the context of contemporary optimal medical care and the ever-expanding and improving array of endovascular techniques. The Claudication versus Endoluminal Revascularization (CLEVER) trial is an ongoing multicenter randomized clinical trial sponsored by the National Heart, Lung, and Blood Institute of the National Institutes of Health comparing supervised exercise to endovascular revascularization for the treatment of claudication due to aortoiliac disease.[84] The results of this ongoing trial will be critical and will likely definitively establish the future standard of care for the treatment of claudication due to aortoiliac disease.

A recent trial from the Netherlands with a design similar to CLEVER randomized 151 patients with claudication to either endovascular revascularization (angioplasty with conditional stenting) or 24 weeks of twice weekly 30-minute hospital-based treadmill exercise sessions.[85] Whereas CLEVER focuses on aortoiliac disease, the Dutch study included patients with iliac or femoral-popliteal disease. They found that endovascular revascularization provided more immediate clinical success but after 6 and 12 months, the treatment groups were equivalent in terms of functional capacity and quality of life scores.[85]

The exact mechanism for the benefits of exercise training on claudication symptoms is not known but is likely multifactorial. Initial theories held that exercise would increase collateral vessels by angiogenesis or lead to increased blood flow but data on these hypotheses are inconsistent.[79,86] Current theory focuses more on changes in muscle metabolism. Potential explanations include metabolic adaptations with improved oxygen extraction by the muscle, better walking efficiency from a biomechanical standpoint, and enhanced endothelial function.[79,87] Hiatt and colleagues,[86] for example, suggest that calf skeletal muscle may increase its oxidative capacity; improvements in exercise correlated with changes in carnitine metabolism.

The benefit of exercise may not be fully explained by local effects on the lower extremities, as evidenced by a recent randomized trial in which 104 patients with PAD were assigned to either upper limb aerobic exercise, lower limb aerobic exercise, or no exercise for 24 weeks.[88] Similar improvements in claudication distance and maximum walking distance were observed in both exercise groups but not in the control group. These results suggest a systemic physiologic benefit of exercise; the investigators also observed an increase in exercise pain tolerance in the exercise groups.

Exercise may also attenuate the inflammatory response over the long-term[79] and has a beneficial effect on cardiovascular risk factors such as hypertension, diabetes, dyslipidemia, and obesity. Further rigorous investigation is needed to ascertain whether this global improvement in vascular health may translate into reduced morbidity or mortality in patients with PAD. A recent retrospective cohort study from

Japan showed that completion of a 12-week supervised exercise training program reduced cardiovascular morbidity and mortality in patients with PAD.[89] Future prospective studies are required to determine the effect of exercise on long-term outcomes in PAD patients.

The efficacy of exercise training for the treatment of symptomatic PAD has been well-established, but recent evidence suggests that exercise training may also play an important role in the treatment of asymptomatic PAD. McDermott and colleagues[87] found that supervised treadmill training improved outcomes (including 6-minute walk performance, treadmill walking performance, and quality of life) not only in patients with claudication but also in patients with PAD who were considered asymptomatic. The same study showed that lower extremity resistance (strength) training was also beneficial in terms of improving functional performance but not to the same degree as supervised treadmill training.[87] This landmark study may herald a change in the approach to the management of asymptomatic PAD; further research in this area is warranted.

BARRIERS TO PAD REHABILITATION

Despite the numerous studies demonstrating the efficacy of exercise training, several barriers prevent the widespread application of this treatment. Most notably, supervised exercise training is not generally covered by third-party payers. PAD rehabilitation has had a Current Procedural Terminology code (CPT 93,668) since 2001, but is generally not a covered benefit by most insurers including Medicare. Most patients are unwilling or unable to pay for a formal program which can cost up to $140 per session; attending 3 sessions per week for 12 weeks could cost more than $5000.

In addition to the financial burden, other barriers to participation include the significant time commitment (for the 30–60 minute sessions and for travel time) and patient compliance. The lack of availability of adequate PAD rehabilitation centers remains a major issue. Barriers may also be at the provider level. For example, a provider may choose not to refer a high-risk patient with multiple comorbidities to an exercise program. Although the provider may hesitate to refer a patient at high cardiovascular risk, that same patient may actually derive the greatest benefit from exercise and may in fact qualify for cardiac rehabilitation as a covered benefit.

Current guidelines[90] outlining appropriate patients for cardiac rehabilitation are in agreement with current coverage under Centers for Medicare and Medicaid Services. At present, cardiac rehabilitation is recommended and generally covered for appropriate patients who have met 1 of the following criteria (effective 3/22/2006):

1. A documented acute myocardial infarction in the preceding 12 months
2. Coronary revascularization including coronary artery bypass surgery or percutaneous transluminal coronary angioplasty
3. Stable angina
4. Heart or lung transplant
5. Heart valve repair or replacement

Unfortunately, cardiac rehabilitation is also historically underutilized by physicians. Only 10% to 20% of eligible patients currently take advantage of formal cardiac rehabilitation programs.[91] Due to the systemic nature of atherosclerotic vascular disease and high prevalence of CAD in this population, in many cases patients with PAD may qualify for cardiac rehabilitation.

The decision to enroll a patient in an exercise training program should be individualized and may be affected by medical comorbidities which limit walking ability. For example, patients may not be able to participate due to neurologic impairment, pulmonary disease, or degenerative joint disease. Treadmill exercise is not recommended in patients with foot ulcers or CLI. Several organizations have published guidelines on contraindications to exercise testing and exercise training including the AHA/ACC and the American College of Sports Medicine. A summary of potential contraindications is shown in **Box 2**.[92]

CURRENT RECOMMENDATIONS FOR EXERCISE TRAINING

Based on available evidence, the investigators are of the opinion that all patients with PAD should be offered exercise training, preferably within a supervised program. As per the ACC/AHA guidelines, standardized treadmill testing should be performed before initiation of exercise training (Class I, Level of Evidence B) to establish the

---

Box 2
Absolute and relative contraindications to exercise testing

Absolute

- Acute MI (within 2 days)
- High-risk unstable angina
- Uncontrolled cardiac arrhythmias causing symptoms of hemodynamic compromise
- Active endocarditis
- Symptomatic severe aortic stenosis
- Decompensated symptomatic heart failure
- Acute pulmonary embolus or pulmonary infarction
- Acute noncardiac disorder that may affect exercise performance or be aggravated by exercise (eg, infection, renal failure, thyrotoxicosis)
- Acute myocarditis or pericarditis
- Physical disability that would preclude safe and adequate test performance
- Inability to obtain consent

Relative[a]

- Left main coronary stenosis or its equivalent
- Moderate stenotic valvular heart disease
- Electrolyte abnormalities
- Tachyarrhythmias or bradyarrhythmias
- Atrial fibrillation with uncontrolled ventricular rate
- Hypertrophic cardiomyopathy
- Mental impairment leading to inability to cooperate
- High-degree AV block

[a] Relative contraindications can be superseded if benefits outweigh risks of exercise.
(*Reprinted from* Fletcher GF, Balady GJ, Amsterdam EA, et al. Exercise standards for testing and training: a statement for healthcare professionals from the American Heart Association. Circulation 2001;104(14):1697, copyright 2001, American Heart Association, Inc; with permission.)

magnitude of the functional limitation due to claudication and to provide a baseline for future comparison to measure the response to therapy.[17] The treadmill test may reveal other nonvascular factors contributing to the impaired walking ability and will help to individualize the exercise prescription. Continuous ECG monitoring is useful, particularly given the high prevalence of CAD in this population. A graded treadmill test is a better tool than a constant-load test because it is more reproducible and shows less variability.[93] For example, the Gardner protocol starts at 2 mph at a 0% grade; the grade is then increased by 2% every 2 minutes.[94] Patients should be instructed to report the onset of claudication symptoms, and the maximum walking time or distance should also be recorded. A 6-minute walk test may be used as an alternative to treadmill testing.[17,87]

The need for cardiac testing before initiation of a formal exercise program should be individualized to the patient. Exercise centers may differ in terms of requirements before enrollment. At minimum, a patient will require a baseline ECG as well as a request from the referring physician. The Johns Hopkins Clinical Exercise Center, for example, requires that patients have a lipid profile, an ECG, recent clinical documentation, as well as a graded exercise test to establish the cardiovascular response to exercise.

The exact nature of the exercise training program differs depending on the center. At present, there are only a limited number of clinical exercise centers in the United States with dedicated PAD rehabilitation programs. Sessions are supervised with monitoring of heart rate and blood pressure; telemetry is typically used for at least the first session and may be used throughout every session if deemed necessary based on the initial response or if requested by the referring physician. Patients with diabetes require blood glucose monitoring to avoid hypoglycemia as exercise increases insulin sensitivity. In addition, proper footwear and routine self-examination of the feet are important, particularly in patients with diabetic neuropathy.

One approach to supervised exercise training as described by Hiatt and colleagues[86] consists of 3 sessions per week for 12 weeks, although more recent studies have employed a 24 week program.[85,87] In Hiatt's program[86] for example, the participant starts with 5 minutes of warm-up, followed by 50 minutes of intermittent exercise, and 5 minutes of cool-down. The intermittent exercise consists of walking on the treadmill starting at 0% grade at 2 mph. The participant walks until the claudication discomfort reaches a moderate level, often described as a "7" on a scale of 1 to 10, preferably within the first 5 minutes on the treadmill. The participant then gets off the treadmill and sits down to rest until the pain subsides completely. As the walking ability increases to 8 to 10 minutes, the grade may be increased by 1 to 2% or the speed may be increased by 0.5 mph as tolerated. The result is multiple intervals of exercise (to near-maximal levels of claudication discomfort) and rest. Participants should also be instructed to walk at home for at least 30 minutes twice per week in addition to the supervised sessions.

Progress in a supervised exercise program can be objectively measured with subsequent treadmill testing, monitoring variables such as pain-free walking time or distance, maximum walking time or distance, or the work performed in metabolic equivalents calculated from the speed and grade of the treadmill. Questionnaires such as the WIQ are not typically used in clinical practice but may be employed as time permits to assess functional status.[93] Repeat testing with ABIs is not generally necessary as the ABI results would not be expected to change[78,81,95] and would not change clinical management as long as the patient continues to progress. As claudication symptoms improve and exercise tolerance increases, patients should be monitored closely for any cardiac signs and symptoms which may have initially been masked by a limited walking ability.

The optimal duration of a supervised exercise program has not been firmly established although 1 would theorize that the longer the program, the better the results. The Gardner and Poehlman meta-analysis found that the best results were seen with walking programs lasting more than 30 minutes per session, at least 3 times per week, for at least 6 months.[57] Studies suggest that the benefits of the supervised program extend beyond the duration of the program. For example, in 1 study of patients who attended supervised training twice weekly for 10 weeks, the improvements in claudication distance and maximum walking distance were sustained at 3 years;[95] there was no difference between the results at 3 months compared with 1, 2, or 3 years.

Following the completion of a supervised program, the patient should be given an exercise prescription to maintain at home using claudication symptoms as a guide. Regular medical follow-up should also be encouraged to optimize medical management focused on cardiovascular risk reduction. Exercise at home should continue with a similar program of intermittent periods of exercise to moderate levels of pain followed by rest until the pain subsides. Several tools may be employed to encourage compliance at home such as follow-up phone calls, using a pedometer, joining a gym, setting goals, keeping a walking diary or logbook, finding an exercise "buddy," and putting daily exercise on a "To-Do List." Web sites such as http://startwalkingnow.org/sponsored by the AHA may be used to plot walking routes and to log walking times and distances.

PAD AWARENESS

Awareness of PAD in general practice is considered a significant issue which may affect the early diagnosis and treatment of these patients. The PARTNERS program was a cross-sectional study aimed at studying the prevalence of PAD in primary care practices in the United States. Using an ABI less than 0.9 to define PAD, the PARTNERS program reported a prevalence of PAD of 29% in patients aged 70 years or older or aged 50 to 69 years with a history of cigarette smoking or diabetes.[5] Most notably, among those patients who were found to have PAD only (exclusive of coronary heart disease), the diagnosis of PAD was new in 55% of patients. In addition, while 83% of patients with prior PAD were aware of their diagnosis, only 49% of their physicians were aware of this diagnosis.[5] Another study aimed at assessing the factors affecting the diagnosis of PAD revealed that only 37% of internists reported taking a history of claudication from their patients; in contrast 92% reported taking a cardiac history most of the time.[96]

Current PAD management guidelines recommend the routine use of ABIs in general medicine practices, specifically in patients who exhibit risk factors for PAD. The most important of those risk factors include: age ≥ 70; age 50 to 69 years with a history of smoking or diabetes; exertional leg symptoms suggestive of claudication; ischemic rest pain; abnormal lower extremity pulse examination; and known atherosclerotic disease.[17] However, the US Preventive Services Task Force currently recommends against routine screening for PAD by ABI testing.[97] Other barriers to the routine use of ABIs such as time constraints, lack of reimbursement, and staff availability have been reported.[98] The Northern Manhattan Study (NOMAS) found that self-reported PAD, defined as a positive answer to 1 of 2 questions related to exertional leg symptoms or a known history of prior PAD, was associated with an independent increased risk of future vascular events in a population-based cohort.[99] Therefore, in the absence of routine use of screening ABIs in general medicine, it would be reasonable to institute questions related to self-reported PAD into the routine medical history. This procedure could lead to an increase in PAD awareness in general practice, increased referral for objective testing, and, ultimately, improved detection of PAD.

It is worthwhile to note that PARTNERS and other studies have reported under-treatment of risk factors in patients with known PAD as compared with patients with CAD.[5,100] Specifically, patients with PAD were less likely to be treated with aspirin and statins than their CAD counterparts.[5,100] These findings highlight the need for increased awareness of PAD in general practice settings, with the goal of training primary care physicians to elicit a history of claudication or atypical leg symptoms in patients considered at high-risk for PAD, so that they may benefit from early diagnosis. This procedure would lead to institution of appropriate early treatment aimed at cardiovascular risk reduction and the use of specific strategies to improve health-related quality of life in patients with PAD.

SUMMARY

The prevalence of PAD is high and will continue to grow with our aging population. It is often underdiagnosed and undertreated due to a general lack of awareness on the part of the patient and the practitioner. The evidence-base is growing for the optimal medical management of the patient with PAD; in parallel, endovascular revascularization options continue to improve. Exercise training for claudication rehabilitation continues to play a critical role. Comprehensive care of the PAD patient focuses on the ultimate goals of improving quality of life and reducing cardiovascular morbidity and mortality.

REFERENCES

1. Belch JJ, Topol EJ, Agnelli G, et al. Critical issues in peripheral arterial disease detection and management: a call to action. Arch Intern Med 2003;163(8): 884–92.
2. Criqui MH, Denenberg JO, Langer RD, et al. The epidemiology of peripheral arterial disease: importance of identifying the population at risk. Vasc Med 1997;2:221–6.
3. Fowkes FGR, Housley E, Cawood EHH, et al. Edinburgh Artery Study: prevalence of asymptomatic and symptomatic peripheral arterial disease in the general population. Int J Epidemiol 1991;20:384–92.
4. Meijer WT, Hoes AW, Rutgers D, et al. Peripheral arterial disease in the elderly: the Rotterdam Study. Arterioscler Thromb Vasc Biol 1998;18:185–92.
5. Hirsch AT, Criqui MH, Treat-Jacobson D, et al. Peripheral arterial disease detection, awareness, and treatment in primary care. JAMA 2001;286:1317–24.
6. Murabito JM, Evans JC, Larson MG, et al. The ankle-brachial index in the elderly and risk of stroke, coronary disease, and death: the Framingham Study. Arch Intern Med 2003;163:1939–42.
7. Ouriel K. Peripheral arterial disease. Lancet 2001;358:1257–64.
8. Ouriel K, McDonnell AE, Metz CE, et al. A critical evaluation of stress testing in the diagnosis of peripheral vascular disease. Surgery 1982;91:686–93.
9. Yao ST, Hobbs JT, Irvine W. Ankle systolic pressure measurements in arterial disease affecting the lower extremities. Br J Surg 1969;59:676–9.
10. Fowkes FG. The measurement of atherosclerotic peripheral arterial disease in epidemiologic surveys. Int J Epidemiol 1988;17:248–54.
11. Feigelson HS, Criqui MH, Fronek A, et al. Screening for peripheral arterial disease: the sensitivity, specificity, and predictive value of noninvasive tests in a defined population. Am J Epidemiol 1994;140:526–34.

12. Criqui MH, Fronek A, Barrett-Connor E, et al. The prevalence of peripheral arterial disease in a defined population. Circulation 1985;71:510–5.
13. Selvin E, Erlinger TP. Prevalence of and risk factors for peripheral arterial disease in the United States. Results from the National Health and Nutrition Examination Survey 1999–2000. Circulation 2004;110:738–43.
14. McDermott MM, Liu K, Criqui MH, et al. Ankle-brachial index and subclinical cardiac and carotid disease. The multi-ethnic study of atherosclerosis. Am J Epidemiol 2005;162:33–41.
15. Morrissey NJ, Giacovelli J, Egorova N, et al. Disparities in the treatment and outcome of vascular disease in Hispanic patients. J Vasc Surg 2007;46:971–8.
16. Norgren L, Hiatt WR, Dormandy JA, et al. on behalf of the TASC-II Working Group. Inter-Society Consensus for the Management of Peripheral Arterial Disease (TASC-II). J Vasc Surg 2007;45(Suppl S):S5–67.
17. Hirsch AT, Haskal ZJ, Hertzer NR, et al. ACC/AHA 2005 guidelines for the management of patients with peripheral arterial disease (lower extremity, renal, mesenteric, and abdominal aortic): executive summary a collaborative report from the American Association for Vascular Surgery/Society for Vascular Surgery, Society for Cardiovascular Angiography and Interventions, Society for Vascular Medicine and Biology, Society of Interventional Radiology, and the ACC/AHA Task Force on Practice Guidelines (Writing Committee to Develop Guidelines for the Management of Patients with Peripheral Arterial Disease) endorsed by the American Association of Cardiovascular and Pulmonary Rehabilitation; National Heart, Lung, and Blood Institute; Society for Vascular Nursing; TransAtlantic Inter-Society Consensus; and Vascular Disease Foundation. J Am Coll Cardiol 2006;47:1239–312.
18. Price JF, Mowbray PI, Lee AJ, et al. Relationship between smoking and cardiovascular risk factors in the development of peripheral arterial disease and coronary artery disease: Edinburgh Artery Study. Eur Heart J 1999;20:344–53.
19. Newman AB, Siscovick DS, Manolio TA, et al. Ankle-arm index as a marker of atherosclerosis in the Cardiovascular Health Study. Cardiovascular Heart Study (CHS) Collaborative Research Group. Circulation 1993;88:837–45.
20. Leng GC, Fowkes FG. The Edinburgh Claudication Questionnaire: an improved version of the WHO/Rose Questionnaire for use in epidemiological surveys. J Clin Epidemiol 1992;45:1101–9.
21. Criqui MH, Fronek A, Klauber MR, et al. The sensitivity, specificity, and predictive value of traditional clinical evaluation of peripheral arterial disease: results from noninvasive testing in a defined population. Circulation 1985;71:516–22.
22. Criqui MH, Denenberg JO, Bird CE, et al. The correlation between symptoms and non-invasive test results in patients referred for peripheral arterial disease testing. Vasc Med 1996;1:65–71.
23. McDermott MM, Greenland P, Liu K, et al. Leg symptoms in peripheral arterial disease: associated clinical characteristics and functional impairment. JAMA 2001;286:1599–606.
24. McDermott MM, Ferrucci L, Simonsick EM, et al. The ankle brachial index and change in lower extremity functioning over time: the Women's Health and Aging Study. J Am Geriatr Soc 2002;50:238–46.
25. Hiatt WR. Drug therapy: medical treatment of peripheral arterial disease and claudication. N Engl J Med 2001;344:1608–21.
26. CAPRIE Steering Committee. A randomised, blinded, trial of clopidogrel versus aspirin in patients at risk of ischaemic events (CAPRIE). Lancet 1996;348:1329–39.

27. Hayoz D, Bounameaux H, Canova CR. Swiss Atherothrombosis Survey: a field report on the occurrence of symptomatic and asymptomatic peripheral arterial disease. J Intern Med 2005;258:238–43.

28. Bhatt DL, Steg GP, Ohman EM, et al. International prevalence, recognition, and treatment of cardiovascular risk factors in outpatients with atherothrombosis. JAMA 2006;295:180–9.

29. Kannel WB, Skinner JJ, Schwartz MJ, et al. Intermittent claudication: incidence in the Framingham Study. Circulation 1970;41:875–83.

30. Criqui MH, Langer RD, Fronek A, et al. Mortality over a period of 10 years in patients with peripheral arterial disease. N Engl J Med 1992;326:381–6.

31. Abbott RD, Rodriguez BL, Pretrovich H, et al. Ankle-brachial blood pressure in elderly men and the risk of stroke: the Honolulu Heart Program. J Clin Epidemiol 2001;54:973–8.

32. Resnick H, Lindsay R, McDermott MM, et al. Relationship of high and low ankle brachial index to all-cause and cardiovascular disease mortality. Circulation 2004;109:733–9.

33. McDermott MM, Liu K, Greenland P, et al. Functional decline in peripheral arterial disease: associations with the ankle brachial index and leg symptoms. JAMA 2004;292:453–61.

34. Khan NA, Rahim SA, Anand SS, et al. Does the clinical examination predict lower extremity peripheral arterial disease? JAMA 2006;295:536–46.

35. Hirsch AT. Arterial occlusive disease of the extremities. In: Creager MA, editor. Atlas of vascular disease. 2nd edition. Philadelphia: Current Medicine, Inc.; 2003. p. 47–79.

36. Rubin GD, Schmidt AJ, Logan LJ, et al. Multi-detector row CT angiography of lower extremity arterial inflow and runoff: initial experience. Radiology 2001; 222:146–58.

37. Owen RS, Carpenter JP, Baum RA, et al. Magnetic resonance imaging of angiographically occult runoff vessels in peripheral arterial occlusive disease. N Engl J Med 1992;326:1577–81.

38. Marckmann P, Skov L, Rossen K, et al. Nephrogenic systemic fibrosis: suspected etiological role of gadodiamide used for contrast-enhanced magnetic resonance imaging. J Am Soc Nephrol 2006;17:2359–62.

39. Jacoby DS, Mohler ER III. Peripheral arterial disease: Risk factor identification and modification. In: Abela GS, editor. Peripheral vascular disease: basic diagnostics and therapeutic approaches. Philadelphia: Lippincott Williams & Wilkins; 2004. p. 190–9.

40. Antithrombotic Trialists' Collaboration. Collaborative meta-analysis of randomised trials of antiplatelet therapy for prevention of death, myocardial infarction, and stroke in high-risk patients. BMJ 2002;324:71–86.

41. Gardner AW. The effect of cigarette smoking on exercise capacity in patients with intermittent claudication. Vasc Med 1996;1(3):181–6.

42. Hurt RD, Sachs DP, Glover ED, et al. A comparison of sustained-release bupropion and placebo for smoking cessation. N Engl J Med 1997;337(17):1195–202.

43. Gonzalez D, Rennard SI, Nides M, et al. Varenicline, an alpha4beta2 nicotinic acetylcholine receptor partial agonist, vs sustained-release bupropion and placebo for smoking cessation: a randomized controlled trial. JAMA 2006;296: 47–55.

44. Jorenby DE, Hays JT, Rigotti NA, et al. Efficacy of varenicline, an alpha4beta2 nicotinic acetylcholine receptor partial agonist, vs placebo or sustained-release

bupropion for smoking cessation: a randomized controlled trial. JAMA 2006;296: 56–63.

45. Available at: http://www.fda.gov/cder/drug/advisory/varenicline.htm. Accessed March 24, 2009.

46. Lee AJ, MacGregor AS, Hau CM, et al. The role of haematologic factors in diabetic peripheral arterial disease: the Edinburgh Artery Study. Br J Haematol 1999;105:648–54.

47. Jude EB, Oyibo SO, Chalmers N, et al. Peripheral arterial disease in diabetic and nondiabetic patients. Diabetes Care 2001;24:1433–7.

48. UK Prospective Diabetes Study Group. The UK Prospective Diabetes Study. Lancet 1998;352:837–53.

49. Hiatt WR, Hoag S, Hamman RF. Effect of diagnostic criteria on the prevalence of peripheral arterial disease. The San Luis Valley Diabetes Study. Circulation 1995;91(5):1472–9.

50. Heart Protection Study Collaborative Group. MRC/BHF Heart Protection Study of cholesterol lowering with simvastatin in 20,536 high-risk individuals: a randomised placebo-controlled trial. Lancet 2002;360:7–22.

51. Pedersen TR, Kjekshus J, Pyorala K, et al. Effect of simvastatin on ischemic signs and symptoms in the Scandinavian simvastatin survival study (4S). Am J Cardiol 1998;81:333–5.

52. Grundy SM, Cleeman JI, Bairey Merz CN, et al. Implications of recent clinical trials for the National Cholesterol Education Program Adult Treatment Panel III guidelines. Circulation 2004;110:227–39.

53. Mehler PS, Coll JR, Estacio R, et al. Intensive blood pressure control reduces the risk of cardiovascular events in patients with peripheral arterial disease and type 2 diabetes. Circulation 2003;107:753–6.

54. Radack K, Deck C. Beta-adrenergic blocker therapy does not worsen intermittent claudication in subjects with peripheral arterial disease: a meta-analysis of randomized controlled trials. Arch Intern Med 1991;151:1769–76.

55. Yusuf S, Sleight P, Pogue J, et al. Effects of an angiotensin-converting-enzyme inhibitor, ramipril, on cardiovascular events in high-risk patients. The Heart Outcomes Prevention Evaluation Study Investigators. N Engl J Med 2000;342:145–53.

56. The ONTARGET Investigators. Telmisartan, ramipril, or both in patients at high risk for vascular events. N Engl J Med 2008;358:1547–59.

57. Gardner AW, Poehlman ET. Exercise rehabilitation programs for the treatment of claudication pain: a meta-analysis. JAMA 1995;274:975–80.

58. Strandness DE Jr, Dalman RL, Panian S, et al. Effect of cilostazol in patients with intermittent claudication: a randomized, double-blind, placebo-controlled study. Vasc Endovascular Surg 2002;36:83–91.

59. Dawson DL, Cutler BS, Meissner MH, et al. Cilostazol has beneficial effects in treatment of intermittent claudication: results from a multicenter, randomized, prospective, double-blind trial. Circulation 1998;98:678–86.

60. Money SR, Herd JA, Isaacsohn JL, et al. Effect of cilostazol on walking distances in patients with intermittent claudication caused by peripheral vascular disease. J Vasc Surg 1998;27:267–74.

61. Beebe HG, Dawson DL, Cutler BS, et al. A new pharmacologic treatment for intermittent claudication: results of a randomized, multicenter trial. Arch Intern Med 1999;159:2041–50.

62. Dawson DL, Cutler BS, Hiatt WR, et al. A comparison of cilostazol and pentoxifylline for treating intermittent claudication. Am J Med 2000;109:523–30.

63. Regensteiner JG, Ware JE Jr, McCarthy WJ, et al. Effect of cilostazol on treadmill walking, community-based walking ability, and health-related quality of life in patients with intermittent claudication due to peripheral arterial disease: meta-analysis of six randomized controlled trials. J Am Geriatr Soc 2002;50:1939–46.

64. Packer M, Carver JR, Rodeheffer RJ, et al. Effect of milrinone on mortality in severe chronic heart failure. N Engl J Med 1991;325:1468–75.

65. Porter JM, Cutler BS, Lee BY, et al. Pentoxifylline efficacy in the treatment of intermittent claudication: multicenter controlled double-blind trial with objective assessment of chronic occlusive peripheral arterial disease patients. Am Heart J 1982;104:66–72.

66. Girolami B, Bernardi E, Prins MH, et al. Treatment of intermittent claudication with physical training, smoking cessation, pentoxifylline, or nafronyl: a meta-analysis. Arch Intern Med 1999;159:337–45.

67. Hood SC, Moher D, Barber GG. Management of intermittent claudication with pentoxifylline: meta-analysis of randomized controlled trials. CMAJ 1996;155:1053–9.

68. Lievre M, Morand S, Besse B, et al. Oral beraprost sodium, a prostaglandin I(2) analogue, for intermittent claudication: a double-blind, randomized, multicenter controlled trial. Beraprost et Claudication Intermittente (BERCI) Research Group. Circulation 2000;102:426–31.

69. Mohler ER 3rd, Hiatt WR, Olin JW, et al. Treatment of intermittent claudication with beraprost sodium, an orally active prostaglandin I2 analogue: a double-blinded, randomized, controlled trial. J Am Coll Cardiol 2003;41:1679–86.

70. Yang HT, Deschenes MR, Ogilvie RW, et al. Basic fibroblast growth factor increases collateral blood flow in rats with femoral arterial ligation. Circ Res 1996;76:62–9.

71. McDermott MM, Greenland P, Ferrucci L, et al. Lower extremity performance is associated with daily life physical activity in individuals with and without peripheral arterial disease. J Am Geriatr Soc 2002;50(2):247–55.

72. Expert Panel on Detection, Evaluation, and Treatment of High Blood Cholesterol in Adults. Executive Summary of The Third Report of The National Cholesterol Education Program (NCEP) Expert Panel on Detection, Evaluation, and Treatment of High Blood Cholesterol in Adults (Adult Treatment Panel III). JAMA 2001;285:2486–97.

73. Gardner AW, Montgomery PS, Parker DE. Metabolic syndrome impairs physical function, health-related quality of life, and peripheral circulation in patients with intermittent claudication. J Vasc Surg 2006;43:1191–7.

74. Diabetes Prevention Program Research Group. Reduction in the incidence of type 2 diabetes mellitus by changes in lifestyle among subjects with impaired glucose tolerance. N Engl J Med 2001;344:1343–50.

75. Erb W. Über das "intermitterende Hinken" und adere nervöse Storungen in Folge von Gefässerkrankungen. [About intermittent walking and nerve disturbances due to vascular disease]. Deutsch Z Nervenheilk 1898;13:1–76 [in German].

76. Larsen OA, Lassen NA. Effect of daily muscular exercise in patients with intermittent claudication. Lancet 1966;2(7473):1093–6.

77. Robeer GG, Brandsma JW, van den Heuvel SP, et al. Exercise therapy for intermittent claudication: a review of the quality of randomised clinical trials and evaluation of predictive factors. Eur J Vasc Endovasc Surg 1998;15:36–43.

78. Watson L, Ellis B, Leng GC. Exercise for intermittent claudication. Cochrane Database Syst Rev 2008;4:CD000990.

79. Stewart KJ, Hiatt WR, Regensteiner JG, et al. Exercise training for claudication. N Engl J Med 2002;347(24):1941–51.

80. Bendermacher BL, Willigendael EM, Teijink JA, et al. Supervised exercise therapy versus non-supervised exercise therapy for intermittent claudication. Cochrane Database Syst Rev 2006;(2):CD005263.

81. Creasy TS, McMillan PJ, Fletcher EWL, et al. Is percutaneous transluminal angioplasty better than exercise for claudication? Preliminary results from a prospective randomized trial. Eur J Vasc Surg 1990;4:135–40.

82. Perkins JMT, Collin J, Creasy TS, et al. Exercise training versus angioplasty for stable claudication. Long and medium term results of a prospective, randomised trial. Eur J Vasc Endovasc Surg 1996;11:409–13.

83. Whyman MR, Fowkes FG, Kerracher EM, et al. Is intermittent claudication improved by percutaneous transluminal angioplasty? A randomized controlled clinical trial. J Vasc Surg 1997;26:551–7.

84. Murphy TP, Hirsch AT, Ricotta JJ, et al. The Claudication: Exercise Vs. Endoluminal Revascularization (CLEVER) study: rationale and methods. J Vasc Surg 2008;47(6):1356–63.

85. Spronk S, Bosch JL, den Hoed PT, et al. Intermittent claudication: clinical effectiveness of endovascular revascularization versus supervised hospital-based exercise training – randomized controlled trial. Radiology 2009;250(2): 586–95.

86. Hiatt WR, Regensteiner JG, Hargarten ME, et al. Benefit of exercise conditioning for patients with peripheral arterial disease. Circulation 1990;81(2):602–9.

87. McDermott MM, Ades P, Guralnik JM, et al. Treadmill exercise and resistance training in patients with peripheral arterial disease with and without intermittent claudication. JAMA 2009;301(2):165–74.

88. Zwierska I, Walker RD, Choksy SA, et al. Upper- vs lower-limb aerobic exercise rehabilitation in patients with symptomatic peripheral arterial disease: a randomized controlled trial. J Vasc Surg 2005;42:1122–30.

89. Sakamoto S, Yokoyama N, Tamori Y, et al. Patients with peripheral artery disease who complete 12-week supervised exercise training program show reduced cardiovascular mortality and morbidity. Circ J 2009;73(1):167–73.

90. Thomas RJ, King M, Lui K, et al. AACVPR/ACC/AHA 2007 performance measures on cardiac rehabilitation for referral to and delivery of cardiac rehabilitation/secondary prevention services endorsed by the American College of Chest Physicians, American College of Sports Medicine, American Physical Therapy Association, Canadian Association of Cardiac Rehabilitation, European Association for Cardiovascular Prevention and Rehabilitation, Inter-American Heart Foundation, National Association of Clinical Nurse Specialists, Preventive Cardiovascular Nurses Association, and the Society of Thoracic Surgeons. J Am Coll Cardiol 2007;50(14):1400–33.

91. Gurewich D, Prottas J, Bhalotra S, et al. System-level factors and use of cardiac rehabilitation. J Cardiopulm Rehabil Prev 2008;28(6):380–5.

92. Fletcher GF, Balady GJ, Amsterdam EA, et al. Exercise standards for testing and training: a statement for healthcare professionals from the American Heart Association. Circulation 2001;104(14):1694–740.

93. Hiatt WR, Hirsch AT, Regensteiner JG, et al. Clinical trials for claudication: assessment of exercise performance, functional status, and clinical endpoints. Circulation 1995;92:614–21.

94. Gardner AW, Skinner JS, Cantwell BW, et al. Progressive vs single-stage treadmill tests for evaluation of claudication. Med Sci Sports Exerc 1991;23: 402–8.

95. Ratliff DA, Puttick M, Libertiny G, et al. Supervised exercise training for intermittent claudication: lasting benefit at three years. Eur J Vasc Endovasc Surg 2007; 34:322–6.

96. McLafferty RB, Dunnington GL, Mattos MA, et al. Factors affecting the diagnosis of peripheral vascular disease before vascular surgery referral. J Vasc Surg 2000;31(5):870–9.

97. United States Preventive Services Task Force. Recommendation statement: screening for peripheral arterial disease. Washington, DC: Agency for Healthcare Research and Quality; 2005. p. 1–8.

98. Mohler ER, Jacobson-Treat D, Reilly MP, et al. Utility and barriers to performance of the ankle-brachial index in primary care practice. Vasc Med 2004;9(4): 253–60.

99. Salameh MJ, Rundek T, Boden-Albala B, et al. Self-reported peripheral arterial disease predicts future vascular events in a community-based cohort. J Gen Intern Med 2008;23:1423–8.

100. McDermott MM, Mehta S, Ahn H, et al. Atherosclerotic risk factors are less intensively treated in patients with peripheral arterial disease than in patients with coronary artery disease. J Gen Intern Med 1997;12:209–15.

Clinical Features and Electrodiagnosis of Diabetic Peripheral Neuropathy in the Dysvascular Patient

Karen Wooten, MD[a,b,]*

KEYWORDS

- Neuropathy • Electrodiagnosis • Diabetes • Dysvascular
- Amputee • Diabetic peripheral neuropathy • Polyneuropathy

Diabetic peripheral neuropathy (DPN) is a common disorder that can lead to limb loss and death. DPN is the most common form of peripheral neuropathy and one of the most common diseases affecting the nervous system. DPN affects greater than half of diabetic patients with a history of more than 25 years of diabetes.[1] There are estimated to be more that 100 million people worldwide with diabetes.[2] One article loosely approximates the United States prevalence of DPN at approximately 7 million patients.[3]

Up to 50% of DPN patients can be asymptomatic, a fact that places such insensate patients who are unaware of their condition at special risk for injuring their feet.[4] This situation contributes to making DPN the leading cause of lower limb amputation.[1] DPN increases the risk of amputation 1.7-fold.[3] Greater than 80% of amputations are related to a foot ulcer or injury.[4] Finally DPN, when accompanied by autonomic neuropathy, increases the chances of death by 25% to 50% within 5 to 10 years.[3] The degree of heterogeneity in the clinical manifestations of DPN and the difficulty involved in diagnosing this condition make for a dangerous combination.

DPN is a very complex disease. This article discusses eight different manifestations of DPN and more than five different tests to help with diagnosis. The diagnosis of DPN is difficult to make. The stakes are high with the large degree of complications associated with DPN.[5] DPN can present to a large number of specialties, ranging from dermatology to podiatry. The main providers for DPN patients are usually

[a] Rehabilitative Care Services (S-117-RCS), Veterans Affairs Puget Sound Health Care System, 1660 S. Columbian Way, Seattle WA 98108, USA
[b] Department of Rehabilitation Medicine, University of Washington, Seattle WA, USA
* Corresponding author. Rehabilitative Care Services (S-117-RCS), Veterans Affairs Puget Sound Health Care System, 1660 S. Columbian Way, Seattle WA 98108, USA.
E-mail address: Karen.wooten@va.gov

Phys Med Rehabil Clin N Am 20 (2009) 657–676
doi:10.1016/j.pmr.2009.06.011
1047-9651/09/$ – see front matter. Published by Elsevier Inc.

diabetologists. Llewelyn points out in his review that neurologists are getting a skewed view of DPN because they are not clinically seeing the full spectrum of DPN.[6] The same could be applied to many physiatrists. To reveal the full clinical spectrum, this article reviews the characteristics, diagnosis, electrodiagnosis, classification, pathogenesis, and treatment of DPN.

CLINICAL CHARACTERISTICS
Definition

Although there are several different types of DPN, this article focuses on the most common type, namely, distal symmetric polyneuropathy (DSPN). The definition of DPN for clinical practice is "the presence of symptoms and/or signs of peripheral nerve dysfunction in people with diabetes after the exclusion of other causes." This definition highlights the important distinction that up to 10% of neuropathies in diabetics can be caused by other things than DPN.[7] There are various risk factors that have been linked with DPN including height, weight, gender, age, disease duration, glycemic control, high blood pressure, tobacco use, alcohol use, and lipids.[8] One of the most interesting of these risk factors is height, specifically tallness. The odds ratio for DPN increases 1.2 for every 10 cm of height,[9] reflecting the length-dependent nature of DPN.

Symptoms

Many of the symptoms of DPN contribute to the cascade that leads to limb loss. Symptoms include pain, weakness, unsteadiness, ataxia, and falls. Some of the most prominent changes occur to sensation.[9] Pain is the most frequently experienced symptom. Pain can be experienced as burning, electrical, deep aching, or stabbing. Often the pain is worse at night. The symptoms are experienced mainly in the feet and lower limbs. When the symptoms get above the ankles or even to the knees, the hands can become involved.[4] Neuropathic sensory changes include the loss of proprioception, pain, and temperature. These changes can increase the risk of trauma, infection, and foot ulceration. Loss of vibration perception places patients at 15 times greater risk of falling.[9]

Unsteadiness was not previously recognized as a feature of DPN. Of late, it has been acknowledged as a legitimate symptom in the literature. Unsteadiness occurs because of changes in lower limb proprioception. Abnormal muscle sensory function also contributes to unsteadiness. This state leads to repetitive trauma and falls that can add to the limb loss cascade.[7] Another cause of falls is "intrinsic minus" muscle wasting in the hands and feet. These changes in the foot lead to unopposed strength in the long toe extensors, resulting in hammertoe deformities. Deformities in the feet increase the risk of ulceration. In addition, poor blood flow from vascular changes compromises wound healing further, increasing the risk of amputation.[9]

Many of the symptoms of DPN can be divided into large fiber versus small fiber. Large fiber changes include weakness, deformities, loss of proprioception, and wasting of small muscles. Small fiber changes include decreased sweating, loss of pain and temperature sensation, dryness of skin, and decreased cutaneous blood flow. All these changes lead to ataxia, falls, fractures, repetitive trauma, deformed joints, ulcerations, and amputations.[6,9]

As pain is the most common symptom, it is worth further exploration. Many words have been used to describe the variety of sensations experienced by patients with DPN. In contrast, some patients have difficulty putting words to their pain and paresthesias. It is important for clinicians to record patients' own words regarding their experience. There are several screening questionnaires that can help capture and define the pain experience of patients with DPN, such as the Michigan Neuropathy Screening Instrument, the visual analog scale, and the NeuroQoL (Neuro Quality of Life).[7]

Sensory symptoms can be divided into positive and negative sensory symptoms. Positive symptoms occur in response to some stimulus or spontaneously, whereas negative symptoms are a decreased response to stimuli. Positive symptoms can be further divided into painful and nonpainful. Examples of nonpainful positive sensory symptoms are descriptors such as stiff, thick, or asleep. A descriptor such as prickling appears in both the painful and nonpainful lists. Painful words include squeezing, throbbing, and freezing. Negative symptoms have been described as numbness or a "dead" feeling. Negative symptoms are easy to measure with Quantitative Sensory Testing (QST); this is not the case with positive symptoms.[7,10]

For this reason, the natural history of negative symptoms has been studied more. A significant question is whether patients' symptoms will improve over time. There have been anecdotal reports of patients' pain symptoms improving or remitting. This remission clinically occurs with worsening sensory changes. One of the limitations of studies looking at this specific issue is that acute and chronic pain syndromes are not always treated separately. Measuring negative symptoms with QST allows researchers to quantify sensory symptoms. In particular, researchers can measure the degree of hypoesthesia with QST. One study showed that type 2 diabetics with hypoesthesia progressed little in the early course of DPN. In patients further in their disease course and experiencing more sensory loss, progression of hypoesthesia was increased.[7]

Signs

Signs of DPN show a symmetric sensory loss to all modalities in a distal to proximal distribution.[7] A study by Perkins and colleagues[11] demonstrated this high degree of symmetry in all the nerves commonly tested in nerve conduction studies except the median nerve. As mentioned before, the sensory loss typically starts to include the hands as the length-dependent neuropathy ascends proximally up the lower limb. Ankle deep tendon reflexes are usually absent or diminished. Sometimes in more severe cases the knee reflexes are also absent. Motor weakness is a less prominent symptom compared with the sensory changes. Intrinsic muscle atrophy occurs commonly in the feet and, in more severe cases, in the hands. More prominent motor signs bring the diagnosis of DPN into question, especially if the motor changes are asymmetric.[7] Physical examination signs of this weakness are often seen on dorsiflexion and plantarflexion weakness. The unsteadiness suffered by DPN patients can manifest as a poor performance on the Rhomberg test, tandem gait, or one-foot stand.[9] Autonomic neuropathy manifests in a distal distribution. Examination may reveal warm, dry skin (without evidence of peripheral vascular disease) or a plantar callus in a pressured area.[7] All these physical examination signs contribute to the diagnosis of DPN.

While tests for DPN are discussed in more depth later, it is worth mentioning the nonpowered, handheld devices that are often used in clinical practice to enhance the neurologic examination. These screening devices are often less sensitive than QST, but are inexpensive, simple, and portable. These devices include the Semmes-Weinstein monofilament test, the tuning fork, and the Neurotip.

The best example is the Semmes-Weinstein monofilament test, which consists of a nylon filament that applies a calibrated degree of pressure on the skin when the monofilament buckles. The main monofilament used is called 5.07 and exerts 10 g of force. The 5.07 is usually assessed at multiple points on the foot. Care must be taken about the type of monofilament used because some studies have identified products that are not correctly calibrated to 10 g of force.[7]

The common tuning fork is 128 Hz. This fork is tested at the apex of the big toe and normally distinguishes vibration. The graduated Rydel-Seiffer tuning fork actually visualizes the vibration intensity using an 8-point scale. This tuning fork correlates accurately with QST. Another device called the Neuropen that has a pin on one side and a 10-g monofilament on the other has also been shown to be sensitive for checking nerve function.[7] These three tools assist in discerning the signs of DPN on physical examination.

Staging

DPN can be further characterized by a 4-staging (0–3) system proposed by Dyck. The staging is based on four tests: Neurology Symptoms Score (NSS), Neurologic Disability Score (NDS), Quantitative Autonomic Function Testing (QAFT), and QST. The NSS allows patients to describe symptoms including sensory, motor, and autonomic changes with an abnormal score being greater than 1. The NDS is based on the neurologic examination. A normal score is greater than 6 and based on sensory, motor, and reflex changes. Autonomic function results are based on heart rate change with deep breathing and are described as normal, borderline, or abnormal. QST uses temperature and vibration sensation tested at the big toe. All these measures synthesize into Stage 0, which is no neuropathy; Stage 1 meaning asymptomatic neuropathy; Stage 2 meaning symptomatic neuropathy; and Stage 3 meaning disabling neuropathy. In Stage 3, there are at least 2 abnormalities on the previously described tests, and evidence of disability on the NDS and NSS.[8,12]

A complementary staging system adds clinical characteristics to each stage of Dyck's system. Clinical neuropathy corresponds with Stage 1. In addition, this system divides Stage 1 into 2 categories: chronic painful and acute painful. Chronic painful is characterized by burning, shooting, and stabbing pains that are increased at night, with reduced or absent reflexes, and absent sensation to multiple modalities. Acute painful has the same symptoms as chronic painful but has few signs on examination and is initiated by changes in insulin therapy. Stage 2 corresponds to painless with complete/partial sensory loss. This stage is defined more by what is not present in symptomatology. There is numbness of the feet or no symptoms, no pain with injury, reduced to absent sensation, absent reflexes, and decreased temperature sensation. Finally, Stage 3 corresponds to late complications that include foot ulceration, joint deformity, and limb loss. Boulton and colleagues[7] suggest that this system adds appropriate clinical modifications to Dyck's staging system (**Table 1**).

DIAGNOSIS
Criteria

The American Academy of Neurology (AAN) has designated five criteria for the diagnosis of DPN. DPN is asymptomatic in many patients and requires multiple tools to diagnose this disease with such prominent complications. The five criteria are symptoms, neurologic examination, electrodiagnostic studies, QST, and autonomic function testing. The AAN recommended that one parameter from each category be tested in the diagnosis of DPN. In clinical practice, two of the five criteria are needed to confirm a diagnosis. Research protocols are more stringent, requiring five out of five categories. The importance of these criteria for the diagnosis of DPN cannot be overemphasized. One study showed that mild DPN was underdiagnosed 62% of the time whereas severe DPN was missed 39% of the time.[13,14]

Table 1		
Dyck's stages of DPN		
Stages of DPN	Description of Neuropathy	Clinical Correlation
1	Asymptomatic	Acute painful
		Chronic painful
2	Symptomatic	Painless with partial or complete sensory loss
3	Disabling	Late complications

Diagnostic Studies

Diagnostic studies including direct biopsy, skin punch biopsy, and QST are reviewed in this section. Studies of more minor importance are discussed together, including magnetic resonance imaging (MRI), confocal corneal microscopy, autonomic testing, and composite measures. The strengths and weaknesses of each test are briefly discussed. Electrodiagnostic studies are discussed in the Section Electrodiagnosis.

Direct biopsy of the nerve has been used to follow the progression of DPN. Direct biopsy is not used routinely for several reasons: it is invasive, can cause sensory deficits, and requires considerable expertise for the analysis. Typically, the sural nerve posterior to the lateral malleolus is sampled. Complications include persistent sensory deficits in the sural distribution and cold intolerance. These complications occur more commonly in diabetics.[7] Direct biopsy of the nerve has mostly been replaced with the skin punch biopsy.

The skin punch biopsy is less invasive, easy, and sensitive. Biopsy technology improved with the discovery of protein gene product 9.5. This gene product is a pan-axonal marker and improves peripheral nerve immunohistologic visualization.[14,15] The typical skin biopsy only requires a 3- to 4-mm diameter sample, sterile technique, and local anesthesia.[2] This technique can look at small nerve fibers, which are difficult to assess in electrodiagnostic studies.[7] Another advantage with punch biopsies is that because there is little trauma, multiple different biopsies can be done, allowing for the examination, if necessary, of different populations of axons especially along a distal to proximal gradient. Punch biopsy is also a good way to monitor progression of DPN. Even with punch biopsies, expertise is still a limitation because only a few centers have the required experience to analyze the biopsy results.[2]

QST pairs well with electrodiagnostic studies. QST can provide information on small fiber changes that are not reflected on nerve conduction studies. QST tests vibration, thermal, and pain thresholds. QST is particularly good at assessing subclinical neuropathy and marking DPN progression.[7] Sima and colleagues suggest that QST, especially vibration and thermal testing combined, should be the primary screening test for DPN. A reduced vibration threshold has been shown to predict for foot ulceration. Thermal testing shows similar predictions. There are several QST devices that are inexpensive, noninvasive, and specific.[13] One recent study showed that vibratory perception testing (VPT) performed on two different instruments yielded equivalent results.[7] Testing with the device takes about 10 minutes for a session. Trained nonmedical personnel can perform this test.[2] The stimulus can be well controlled and can measure a broad range of intensities. QST can be tested at multiple anatomic sites and can track the distal to proximal gradient of DPN. Finally, there is a plethora of data available on normals.

There are a few disadvantages to QST. One limitation is that QST is only semiobjective: it is affected by a patient's motivation, attention, age, sex, and use of tobacco or alcohol.[7] This limitation makes QST unsuitable for assessing patients suspected of malingering or those involved in legal proceedings.[16] QST also is not specific to peripheral nerves. Similar to evoked potentials, it assesses the entire neuroaxis.[7] Abnormal results on QST can be due to spinal cord or cortical lesions.[17] In the 2005 review of the literature by England and colleagues, QST was not found to be reproducible enough to be recommended as the primary criterion for diagnosis of DPN.

Additional Studies

There are several other methods of looking at DPN, one of which is peripheral nerve imaging. MRI of the nerve is noninvasive, targets specific areas, and is easily repeatable. The limits include cost and poorly defined sensitivity. Studies of the sural nerve in diabetics with known DPN and even subacute DPN shows increased water content. This finding indicates endoneurial edema, which reflects early changes that will eventually yield electrodiagnostic changes.[2]

Another suggested method is confocal corneal microscopy, consisting in scanning the cornea for the Bowman layer, which is abundant with a nerve plexus. With microscopy it is easy to examine nerve fiber density, length, and branch density. These nerve characteristics can correlate with progression and severity of DPN. Like MRI, confocal corneal microscopy is noninvasive and might serve a more prominent role in the future.

Quantitative autonomic function testing (QAFT) has been around for a long time. The common tests used for diabetes are based on blood pressure and heart rate response to different maneuvers. Specific tests can assess other affected systems including the urinary, gastrointestinal, and sudomotor. QAFT is included as one of five criteria for the diagnosis of DPN. An in-depth discussion of QAFT is beyond the scope of this article.[14,18]

Composite measures have been developed to integrate all the different tests discussed into the difficult task of diagnosing DPN. There are several different composite measures, the most prominent of which is the Neuropathy Impairment Score in Lower Limbs (NIS-LL). Like the other systems, it provides a single score based on the results of multiple tests. The single score is a percentage of the abnormality. One limitation with relying solely on a composite scoring system is it can mask problems noted on individual tests; another is that composite systems are time consuming in a clinical setting.[17,18]

ELECTRODIAGNOSIS

Electrodiagnostic studies are a fundamental part of diagnosing and assessing DPN. Electrophysiologic testing fits into a larger scheme for diagnosing DPN with tests such as QST, QAFT, and nerve biopsy. Like all tests, it is important to understand the purposes, strengths, weaknesses, and components of electrophysiologic testing.

Purpose

Electrodiagnostic studies have four main purposes: they assess the onset and progression of DPN; evaluate the distribution of a polyneuropathy; rule out other disorders; and serve as an end point in clinical studies to test treatments and pathophysiology.[7,19]

The importance of establishing the diagnosis and assessing the progression of DPN cannot be overstated. DPN is a disease that often has a long subacute phase and is associated with more than half of all limb amputations.[17] DPN is not a reversible condition except through glycemic control. DPN is a disease that shows a disconnection between the development of symptoms and the severity of the pathology. Nerve conduction studies (NCS) are objective, noninvasive, and reliable measures; they are also sensitive and specific to polyneuropathy. For these reasons, electrophysiologic testing is important for establishing the diagnosis and monitoring the progression of DPN.[7,17,20]

Electrophysiologic studies can pinpoint distribution and narrow the differential diagnosis. Electromyography (EMG) and NCS help determine distribution; they differentiate focal from multifocal problems, define symmetry, identify proximal from distal, and demonstrate motor and sensory involvement. NCS can specify the segment of the nerve involved. The tests can also distinguish acute from chronic changes and whether a neuropathy is length dependent.[21] All these factors can help rule out conditions not related to diabetes and define the type of neuropathy involved.

One of the most important roles of electrodiagnosis is to rule out nondiabetic causes of a symmetric polyneuropathy. DPN is a difficult diagnosis to make by itself. There is the added complication that up to 10% of patients diagnosed with DPN have neuropathies from other causes. Electrodiagnostic testing can show whether a patient has chronic inflammatory demyelinating polyneuropathy (CIDP), inflammatory myopathy, motor neuron disease, or other conditions.[7] If DPN shows features of a small fiber polyneuropathy, amyloidosis and lepromatous leprosy should be considered in the differential diagnosis. Amyloidosis is associated with autonomic symptoms, but not leprosy. A nerve biopsy showing nerve thickening can differentiate these two conditions. Vitamin B12 deficiency, paraneoplastic syndrome, and Sjögren's syndrome can present as a pure sensory neuropathy with large fiber involvement. More motor involvement may indicate CIDP or paraproteinemic neuropathy. A nerve biopsy shows inflammation.[12] It is important to identify these conditions because many of them are more treatable than DPN.

Finally, electrodiagnostic studies have helped elucidate pathophysiology and vet treatments. The pathogenesis of DPN is controversial. The major proposed ideas include immunologic changes, metabolic disturbances, or ischemic damage.[22] What is agreed on is the pattern of structural and neural deficits. DPN is characterized as an axonopathy. The cell body remains intact whereas the distal peripheral axon changes.[23] One change in DPN is the alteration of the transmembrane ion gradient. This change disturbs the transduction of neural activity,[7] causing hyperexcitable firing of the nerve that can lead to positive symptoms such as pain and paresthesias. Demyelination occurs in the later stages of DPN. Wallerian degeneration and other changes add to negative symptoms, such as, numbness and weakness.[23] Results of glycemic control can be reflected in the nerve conduction velocity, a component of NCS. Nerve conduction velocity can change with efficacious therapies such as transplantation. All this information adds value to electrophysiologic tests in the assessment of DPN.[7]

Limitations

There are several limitations to the electrodiagnostic testing that are worth highlighting. A weakness of NCS is that the recordings are only taken at the surface, meaning that only a small fraction of the neural activity is measured.[17] Nerve conduction velocity measures mainly large-diameter, heavily myelinated axons,[7] does not show axonopathy well, and reflects the speed of only the largest myelinated fibers. These tests do not reflect changes in the small fibers either.[19] Perkins argues that this is not such a big weakness. He notes that DPN causes a progressive loss of all nerve fibers. Finally, the decreased availability and discomfort of electrodiagnostic studies limits their utility as a screening test.[17]

Evaluation

The goals of an electrodiagnosis evaluation are simple. First, it is important to identify sensory and motor involvement. A full evaluation localizes changes to the motor neuron, nerve root, axon, neuromuscular junction, or muscle fiber. Second, it is necessary to separate axonal degeneration from demyelination. Axonal lesions show reduced amplitudes, little or no changes in nerve conduction velocity, and neurogenic changes on EMG. Conduction slowing mostly reflects demyelination.[20] Standard NCS includes examination of the motor function of peroneal, tibial, median, and ulnar nerves. The sensory function is measured mainly in the sural, median, ulnar, and radial nerves.[17]

Donofrio and Albers lay out a polyneuropathy protocol in the American Academy of Electromyographers minimonograph. These investigators discuss a standard examination including multiple nerves in the upper and lower extremities, both sides, and distal and proximal places. Severity of the disease helps shape the examination. Patients with mild symptoms need the most sensitive or susceptible nerves to be checked.[24] One study found the plantar and sural sensory nerves showed the first indication of early DPN. Sensory and motor nerve amplitudes decline in a nonlinear, distal to proximal fashion as DPN progresses.[17] It is important to take an individual approach to each electrodiagnostic study in assessing DPN.

Components

The components of electrodiagnostic studies include nerve conduction velocity, sensory and motor amplitudes, EMG, F waves, H reflexes, and somatosensory evoked potentials. NCS can give clues about the underlying pathology. Wallerian degeneration demonstrates small changes in amplitude with no changes in nerve conduction velocity. Axonopathy reflects only mild changes in nerve conduction velocity. Demyelination shows changes in the conduction velocity or latency. Conduction block from focal compression shows a sudden drop in amplitude.[21] Nerve conduction parameters such as nerve conduction velocity have revealed much about the natural history of DPN. Nerve conduction velocity decreases very gradually over time.[7] In the early stages of DPN, the maximal conduction velocity changes 0.5 to 0.7 m/s per year, reflecting the lack of demyelination in the early stages of DPN.[2] The sural nerve changes slightly more than the peroneal nerve. Nerve conduction velocity can detect subclinical deficits in DPN in asymptomatic patients.

Progression of DPN can be followed via slight changes in the amplitude and conduction velocity.[21] Symmetry of the nerve abnormalities has been shown to be very important. A study by Perkins and colleagues suggests that if side-to-side differences are more than 10% in DPN, another disease should be considered. The study also suggests unilateral NCS are adequate for following progression of DPN.[11] Amplitudes can correspond to fiber density, but variability in amplitude measures makes it difficult to use amplitude as an early measure of DPN.[2]

EMG can reveal some clues about the timing of the neural changes. Fibrillation potentials can indicate a more acute process. Absence of fibrillation potentials can be seen in a milder, more chronic neuropathy. Somatosensory evoked potentials, F-wave latencies, and H reflexes can show changes proximally. F waves, especially, are sensitive to accumulated changes along the entire length of the nerve. Changes solely in the distal segment might not be well represented with F-wave latencies.[20,25]

CLASSIFICATION

There are multiple ways to classify diabetic neuropathies, ranging from clinical to anatomic. Because the etiology of many of these types of neuropathy is poorly understood, no system is perfect. These systems seek to describe the vast number of neurologic disturbances occurring in nerves from diabetic metabolic and vascular changes.

Bansal and colleagues suggest the main dividing feature is symmetric versus asymmetric neuropathies. Examples of symmetric neuropathies are autonomic neuropathies, diabetic cachexia, diabetic polyneuropathy, CIDP, and diabetic polyneuropathies including those from glucose impairment and ketoacidosis. Asymmetric neuropathies include mononeuropathies, radiculoplexoneuropathies, and cranial neuropathies.[14] Another system divides them into large fiber neuropathy; small fiber neuropathy; proximal motor neuropathy; acute mononeuropathies; and pressure palsies.[3]

Boulton and colleagues refer to three different classification systems. The first continues the clinical theme by dividing neuropathies into polyneuropathies against mononeuropathies. The second describes patterns of neuropathy including length-dependent diabetic polyneuropathy, focal and multiple neuropathies, and nondiabetic neuropathies more common in diabetics (eg, pressure palsies). The final classification adds in the consequence of hyperglycemia, referring to neuropathies not as a single condition but a myriad of conditions affecting the peripheral nervous system. The three main categories of this system are rapidly reversible, generalized symmetric polyneuropathies, and focal and multifocal neuropathies. What follows is a summary of Thomas' system with some modifications (**Table 2**).[7]

Rapidly Reversible Hyperglycemic Neuropathy

Rapidly reversible hyperglycemic neuropathy has been recognized for many years. Rapidly reversible hyperglycemic neuropathy can occur in times of metabolic turbulence such as before the diagnosis of diabetes is established, during times of poor glycemic control, after ketoacidosis, or during changes in glycemic control (also known as insulin neuritis). The most interesting feature of this neuropathy that places it in a separate category is that the symptoms of distal pain are reversible. This feature implies that there is not a structural change in the nerves despite the fact nerve conduction velocity increases. There is a question about whether this can increase one's future risk for developing neuropathy. Sensory symptoms can be severe, remain distal, and are worse at night. Euglycemia reverses the symptoms.[4,7]

Generalized Symmetric Polyneuropathies

Generalized symmetric polyneuropathies include distal symmetric polyneuropathy, autonomic neuropathy (AN), and diabetic cachexia.

Distal symmetric polyneuropathy is by far the most common diabetic neuropathy. As this section reflects, there are many different manifestations of diabetic neuropathy, but distal sensory polyneuropathy can account for two-thirds of the cases.[14]

Table 2 Thomas' modified DPN classification system		
Rapidly Reversible Hyperglycemic Neuropathy	**Generalized Symmetric Polyneuropathy**	**Focal and Multifocal Neuropathies**
—	Chronic sensorimotor neuropathy	Limb mononeuropathy
—	Acute sensory neuropathy	Cranial neuropathy
—	Autonomic neuropathy	Truncal radiculoneuropathy
—	Diabetic cachexia	Proximal motor neuropathy

Distal symmetric polyneuropathy is a length-dependent neuropathy with motor and sensory involvement.[6] The sensory is the most prominent feature, appearing in a stocking and glove distribution. The sensory symptoms usually reach up to the knee before they start in the hands.[14] In severe cases, the sensory changes can extend up to the trunk, first going up the anterior chest and spreading laterally.[6] Motor symptoms are less pronounced.

In addition, distal symmetric polyneuropathy can be divided into small and large fiber neuropathies. These neuropathies mainly represent ends of the spectrum of distal symmetric polyneuropathy, but can be useful to consider clinically because they divide the neuropathy further by sensory modalities.[6] Loss of pain and temperature are associated with small fiber neuropathy. Patients notice more pain and burning sensations. NCS are usually normal. In contrast, large fiber neuropathy impairs touch and pressure sensations, vibration, and joint position. Patients experience painless paresthesias and, in severe forms, sensory ataxia. Nerve conduction velocities are slowed. Distal symmetric polyneuropathy progresses with the loss of ankle reflexes and decreased vibration sensation in the toes. Severe motor symptoms include weakness in toe flexion and extension, and ankle dorsiflexion. Autonomic symptoms can occur at any stage but are more common with severe cases of neuropathy.[21]

Whereas autonomic function tests can show abnormalities in 97% of patients with DPN, AN can be a clinical entity that is not diagnosed quickly.[6] Some investigators add it as part of distal symmetric polyneuropathy, but this classification system treats it as a separate entity. AN affects multiple organ systems including cardiovascular, gastrointestinal, urinary, and metabolic, among others. Most patients experience subclinical manifestations to the cardiovascular and sudomotor systems. Hallmark signs include orthostatic hypertension, unresponsiveness of heart rate to breathing, and resting tachycardia.[14] There are several bedside tests that can be used to test for AN. Tight glycemic control provides some help, but most patients are treated symptomatically. Mortality is increased with AN.[26] Patients with AN suffer from silent myocardial infarctions. One-quarter to half of all AN patients can have their life spans shortened by up to 10 years.[14]

Diabetic neuropathic cachexia is a rare but dramatic manifestation of diabetic neuropathy. Patients are mostly male, though cachexia is occasionally noted in females. The involuntary loss of up to 60% of body weight can be confused with an occult cancer, but the prognosis is positive with symptoms resolving over time. The main symptoms are marked weight loss, emotional problems, symmetric peripheral neuropathy, autonomic dysfunction, and painful paresthesias over the trunk and limbs. The cause remains unknown, but is likely metabolic because the symptoms resolve.[27] Diabetic neuropathic cachexia occurs in men with a mild form of type 2 diabetes, and can be the first signal that someone has developed diabetes or can appear in patients with mild or controlled forms of diabetes. There is a lack of end-organ damage such as retinopathy. This presentation, along with biopsies showing normal vasa nervorum and spontaneous resolution of symptoms, suggests a metabolic mechanism of action versus a microvascular cause.

Diabetic neuropathic cachexia is distinct from other manifestations of diabetic neuropathy. The onset is quick (weeks to months versus years in conventional diabetic neuropathy). The symptoms are severe, peripheral, symmetric, and involve motor and sensory nerves. The most prominent component is painful dysesthesias, sometimes ascending, often involving the proximal limbs and trunk, and worse at night.[28] Sensory symptoms as well as the motor effects can be minimal. There can be muscle atrophy and weakness, but pain is usually the main component of this neuropathy. Treatment for the dysesthesias is symptomatic and reassurance is key.[27] Diabetic cachexia contrasts with diabetic neuropathy in its quick onset, dramatic weight loss, painful dysesthesias, and resolution in 12 to 48 months.[28]

Focal and Multifocal Neuropathies

Focal and multifocal neuropathies are the final category and include mononeuropathies, cranial neuropathies, truncal radiculoneuropathies, proximal motor neuropathies, and CIDP. These neuropathies are more common in type 2 diabetics and thus more relevant to a discussion about dysvascular patients. Diabetics are more likely to develop entrapment syndromes. Specifically, they are at a threefold greater risk for carpal tunnel syndrome.[7]

Limb mononeuropathies occur most commonly in median, ulnar, radial, medial and lateral plantar, lateral femoral cutaneous nerve of the thigh, and peroneal nerves.[7] Common clinical presentations are carpal tunnel syndrome, cubital tunnel syndrome, foot drop, or oculomotor palsy. Mononeuropathies are accompanied by a generalized distal symmetric polyneuropathy, possibly making it difficult to differentiate the mononeuropathies on electrodiagnostics.[22] Median and ulnar neuropathies are the first and second most common mononeuropathies. The treatments and diagnosis of diabetic neuropathies is similar to that of nondiabetic mononeuropathies.[7] Several mononeuropathies appearing in combination at the same time could indicate mononeuritis multiplex.[22] Compression is definitely involved, and nerve infarctions from occlusion of the vasa nervosum can occur. Systemic vasculitis should be ruled out in the case of multiple mononeuropathies.[14]

Cranial neuropathies constitute one of the rarer diabetic neuropathies. Of these, the ocular nerves are more affected than the facial nerve.[7] These cranial nerve palsies affect older patients with diabetes of longer than a year's duration and with evidence of distal symmetric polyneuropathy. The onset is usually abrupt and painless. Oculomotor neuropathy is more common than trochlear or abducens.[14] The third nerve palsy often starts with retro-orbital pain that lasts for a few days. One feature of this palsy is sparing of the pupillary function, as the nerve fibers are peripheral and do not seem to be affected by the ischemia. The sparing of the pupillary function is supposed to be the hallmark of diabetic involvement. Imaging is still needed to rule out a structural lesion such as an aneurysm.[6] Boulton and colleagues[7] cites a study showing that up to 18% of diabetics do develop pupillary dysfunction. In general, these neuropathies are easily diagnosed and self-limited with resolution in a few months to a year.

The final three presentations of focal and multifocal diabetic neuropathies are often bundled together. In Thomas' classification system, they are treated separately under focal and multifocal neuropathies. In other sources, they are categorized as asymmetric proximal diabetic neuropathies.[14]

Diabetic truncal radiculoneuropathy can occur in type 1 or 2 diabetes, start in middle or older age, and have an acute onset; it is not progressive like distal symmetric polyneuropathy, but resembles diabetic cachexia in the way it often remits. The course of this neuropathy is more dramatic, being characterized with focal lancinating pain in the abdomen unilaterally (rarely bilaterally) with hyperesthesias worsened at night.[6] On occasion there is motor involvement with bulging of the abdominal wall. Paresthesias involve the T4 to T12 distribution.[14] Physical examination can reveal changes from no abnormality to sensory loss and hyperesthesia in a dermatomal distribution. Etiology is unknown but is thought to be vascular because of the acute onset and recovery. There does seem to be a metabolic element to the pathogenesis because it is more common in patients with poorer glycemic control. Recovery usually occurs in 4 to 6 months.[7]

The biggest problem with diabetic amyotrophy is that it has an overabundance of names, thus reflecting the ambiguity of the syndrome's clinical characterization and mechanism of action. The eponymous term is Bruns-Garland syndrome.[6] Descriptive terms include diabetic lumbosacral radiculoplexus neuropathy and asymmetric proximal diabetic neuropathy. A simpler terminology that reflects this ambiguity is diabetic proximal neuropathy. All these terms reflect some of the features of this syndrome. A uniting feature is the involvement of a root or proximal nerve.[14]

Diabetic amyotrophy occurs in patients 50 to 60 years old with type 2 diabetes. The clinical picture includes severe pain, unilateral or bilateral muscle weakness, and proximal thigh muscle atrophy.[7] Pain occurs in the lower back, anterior thighs, or buttocks. The weakness can follow within days to weeks of the pain. The distribution is proximal with occasional distal muscle involvement. Patients can even develop generalized leg paresis termed diabetic paraparesis. Weight loss can also occur. The pain and weight loss starts to resolve, but the recovery of the weakness occurs over a longer period spanning months. Unlike diabetic truncal radiculoneuropathy, the loss of strength can linger in some cases. When the presentation appears as unilateral weakness with weight loss, the differential diagnosis should include pelvic malignancy or radiotherapy. If there is no pain with progressive asymmetric leg weakness, CIDP, the last of the proximal diabetic polyneuropathies, should be considered.[6]

It is important to recognize CIDP because of the diabetic polyneuropathies, it is the most treatable. Besides being painless, it is unusually severe and progressive. One important diagnostic feature is the presence of macrophage-associated demyelination on the biopsy. This feature is characteristic of CIDP and is not shared with other diabetic polyneuropathies. CIDP is 11 times more common in diabetics than in the normal population. The treatment is immunomodulation via steroids, intravenous immunoglobulin (IVIG), or plasmapheresis.[7]

PATHOGENESIS

The pathogenesis for DPN is convoluted, complicated, and intimately intertwined with the changes that lead to amputation. The cause of DPN is unknown.[29] As discussed before, the fact DPN is such a heterogeneous disease makes finding the uniting cause difficult.[3] Most efforts are focused on distal symmetric polyneuropathy, the more common form of DPN. The pathogenesis of DPN is multifactorial with the main categories being metabolic and ischemic. In addition, genetic predisposition and environmental factors such as smoking and alcohol use affect the pathogenesis of DPN. The two mechanisms of metabolism and vascular do not have to be thought of as exclusive, but can work together.[29]

Hyperglycemia

The primary metabolic mechanism is persistent hyperglycemia. Hyperglycemia is the best-studied mechanism, as it was the sole treatment option shown to change the course of DPN in the Diabetes Control and Complications Trial (DCCT). The DCCT study showed that controlling blood glucose can decrease the risk of developing DPN by 60% over 5 years. Controlling hyperglycemia is the main clinical means of controlling DPN.[1] Glucose provides the only source of fuel for peripheral nerves; it enters nerve cells and is used in the production of adenosine triphosphate. Glucose enters nerve cells independently of insulin. Myo-inositol is a normal, dietary hexose that is found abundantly in the peripheral nerve, 100 times the concentration of plasma. Hyperglycemia inhibits the normal uptake of myo-inositol because the transport system is busy taking up the abundant glucose, leading to a decrease in the myo-inositol within the nerve. This action prolongs nerve conduction, causing nerve dysfunction.[30]

Long-term hyperglycemia also activates the polyol pathways. The excess glucose is converted to sorbitol by an enzyme called aldose reductase, causing the accumulation of sorbitol in the nerve cell. Sorbitol is metabolized to fructose. The cell can clear neither sorbitol nor fructose.[30] Their accumulation leads to intracellular osmotic stress.[31]

Other consequences of hyperglycemia include oxidative stress and glycation of proteins. Oxidative stress occurs because of the revved-up polyol pathway. When sorbitol and fructose are being produced due to increased intracellular glucose from hyperglycemia, the oxidation/reduction status of the cell is changed, resulting in an increase of free radicals. The free radicals disrupt the nerve cell's proteins and lipids and, thus, disrupt the nerve. This oxidative stress also decreases the nitrous oxide within the small blood vessels supplying the nerve, leading to low nerve blood flow and ischemia. This sequence of events is another example of how the metabolic and vascular mechanisms are entwined.[1,9]

Another hyperglycemic mechanism of DPN mentioned in several other articles is nonenzymatic glycation of proteins. Tomlinson and Gardiner point out that finding out the exact functional and structural impact of glycation has been limited by the lack of treatment for this mechanism. With the polyol pathway discussed previously, aldose reductase inhibitors (ARIs) allow a concrete way to study the pathway. ARIs block the enzyme aldose reductase and stop the changes to the polyol pathway. It is known that glycation causes nerve dysfunction. Not having an adequate treatment molecule such as an ARI has inhibited finding out the exact consequences of glycation. Tomlinson and Gardiner suggest that new glycation inhibitors, such as pyridoxamine, are a promising avenue of research.[31]

Some of the mechanisms of hyperglycemia correspond to the natural history of DPN. Aberrations in glycemic pathways include the formation of sorbitol and fructose, the decrease in intracellular myo-inositol, and the nonenzymatic glycation of proteins. These aberrations seem to be interconnected and also may occur sequentially. Some examples include the change in the polyol pathway occurring early in the course of DPN. In contrast, these changes are not found in the polyol pathway with chronic forms of DPN. Nonenzymatic glycation is more prominent with later progression of DPN. Problems with immune responses occur later in DPN.[13]

Ischemia

Local nerve ischemia contributes to the degeneration of nerves. Sural nerve biopsies have shown local vascular disease changes. These changes include reduced blood flow, basement membrane thickening, endothelial cell proliferation, and vessel occlusion. The nerves themselves develop a primary axonopathy in myelinated and unmyelinated nerves. The process of nerve degeneration is simultaneous with nerve regeneration within the nerve. The processes of nerve degeneration and regeneration can be dynamic, shifting between these 2 states.[1]

Ischemia causes different types of nerve degeneration between diabetes types 1 and 2. Type 2 diabetics differ from type 1 diabetics in that they show milder axonal atrophy with fewer nodal changes. The nerve fiber loss in older type 2 diabetics tends to be more focused, indicating a more vascular cause. Type 2 patients also have a significantly higher frequency of Wallerian degeneration. Type 2 diabetics have a broader range of fibers involved than type 1 diabetics. Type 2 diabetics also have a wider variety of neuropathies caused by diabetes compared with type 1 diabetics.[25] Sima and colleagues report that treatment studies for type 2 diabetics often display more disappointing results than for type 1 diabetics. All these changes indicate that there are different mechanisms of DPN between different types of diabetes. For this reason, type 2 diabetics should have their own focus for clinical trials on treatment.[13]

Microvascular changes cause ischemia and hypoxia at the cellular level. One of the main changes of diabetic microangiopathy is thickening of the basement membrane of capillaries. This thickening also occurs in the kidney and eye. Microvascular changes are related to the duration of diabetes, being seen in 100% of patients with diabetes of more than 20 years' duration. Large vessel changes do not correlate well with progression of DPN. Small vessel changes, on the other hand, link with the severity of DPN. Changes include an increase in number of endothelial cells in the endoneurial capillary. The endoneurial capillary can also become occluded. Segmental loss of myelin fibers might be due to areas of poor perfusion or ischemia.[30] Functional changes include decreased neural blood flow, increased vascular resistance, and changed vascular permeability. Changes in cutaneous blood flow also correlate with DPN.[32] Vascular changes in diabetes reflect the characteristics of DPN. Occurrence of arterial degeneration is of a more distal nature in diabetics. This degeneration increases vessel calcification and increases the risk of infection in diabetic limbs at risk for amputation.[33]

Other Mechanisms

Other less understood mechanisms include immune, genetic, and neurotrophic.[3] Studies of these and most mechanisms use animal models. Animal models used include rodent models such as chemically inducing diabetes type 1 in rats by injecting streptozocin to destroy the pancreatic insulin-producing cells. One of the limitations of these models is that rodents do not exhibit the same pathophysiology or symptomatology as humans. Also, the studies are often too short to model the long-term effects of DPN.[9]

Autoimmune changes have been noted in patients with DPN. Antibodies seem to cause nerve dysfunction, but do not seem to affect blood flow or cause vascular changes. Immune mechanisms have been identified in patients with a more prominent motor component to their neuropathies or in patients with more proximal neuropathies. Multiple studies have shown the presence of antibodies in the serum of diabetic patients with neuropathy. One study showed the presence of antiganglioside antibody in 12% of the tested diabetic patients with DPN. This antibody is associated electrophysiologically with a neuropathy that has a stronger motor component. Other studies have shown immunoglobulins with complement factors facilitating the cell death of neuronal cells in culture. Autoimmunity is a secondary mechanism that could lead to treatment of a smaller constituency of patients with DPN.[9,32]

Another mechanism being investigated is the role of neurotrophic factors. Neurotrophic factors are proteins that promote the survival, maintenance, and regeneration of neurons, especially in the setting of the noxious effects of diabetes. The reduction of neurotrophic factors can cause neuronal loss, likely through apoptosis (programmed cell death). Neurotrophic factors include nerve growth factor (NGF), vascular endothelial growth factor (VEGF), and insulin-like growth factor-1 (IGF-1). NGF is the best studied of these proteins. NGF promotes the survival of sympathetic and small fiber sensory neurons, which are the main neuronal victims of DPN. NGF production has been shown to be impaired in animal studies. The level of NGF in the skin keratinocytes of diabetics correlates with small fiber sensory neuropathy. VEGF is produced when there is ischemia, and promotes increased blood flow through angiogenesis.

VEGF also improves nerve function. Treatment with NGF has been met with limited success. Of note, antioxidant therapy seems to enhance NGF actions.[9,31,32]

TREATMENT

Treatment falls into 2 categories, those affecting pathogenesis and those providing symptomatic treatment. A current understanding of the pathogenesis is important because all of the treatment attempts to stop DPN come from these mechanisms. Treatment needs to bring all these mechanisms of DPN into play. Research has given a good overview of the principal components of pathogenesis, as outlined earlier. Focusing on a single mechanism has not always worked. ARIs, though showing some small improvements in DPN, have not been successful clinically. One reason for this might be that by blocking the polyol pathway, another pathway, glycation, is left open. More glucose might be diverted by the ARIs to the glycation pathway. Combination treatments that block protein glycation with ARIs might be a promising future option. Other mechanisms such as oxidative stress and neurotrophic dysfunction should be explored. Antioxidants, which limit the damage from reactive oxygen species, would likely be helpful. Neurotrophic factors, such as NGF, would also help reduce oxidative stress and also might increase nerve regeneration. Combination therapies are the next focus for research.[1,31]

Pathogenic Treatment

The main and most proven treatment from the study of pathogenesis is near-normoglycemia. The DCCT showed that normoglycemia was the main viable treatment for DPN. One study looked at diabetic patients at the time of diagnosis and then 25 years beyond the diagnosis of diabetes. The study showed that detectable DPN increased from 12% at diagnosis to 50% at 25 years. The highest prevalence of DPN was in the patients with the poorest glycemic control.[14]

Rigid glycemic control can be achieved by multiple daily injections, subcutaneous insulin infusion, or pancreatic transplant. The DCCT did not separate patients receiving multiple injections or subcutaneous insulin infusion. The Oslo study looked specifically at the continuous subcutaneous insulin infusion. The insulin infusion improved motor nerve conduction velocity and sensory nerve action potential amplitudes significantly compared with conventional treatment (insulin injections once or twice a day).[34] The DCCT showed that intensive glycemic control resulted in a decrease of 64% in patients developing DPN after 5 years.[35] Moreover, the study showed that intensive glycemic control was possible, sustainable over 5 years, achievable in lots of different clinical settings, and blunted the presence and progression of DPN.[34]

The DCCT study also revealed the risks of tight glycemic control. Patients with continuous subcutaneous insulin injections were at less risk of severe hypoglycemia, but did suffer from increased asymptomatic hypoglycemia. The DCCT showed that severe hypoglycemic episodes were three times higher in patients practicing tight glycemic control. Although not seen in the study, recurrent hypoglycemia over a lifetime may result in progressive cognitive problems.

There are several limitations with the pivotal DCCT study. First, the investigators used surrogate measures instead of more direct measures such as quality of life or complication rate. Second, study patients mostly had mild DPN or even asymptomatic DPN, meaning that the DCCT results do not address the issues related to advanced neuropathy. Third, both arms of the study focused on type 1 diabetics. In addition, because the DCCT excluded all other types of diabetic neuropathies such as diabetic amyotrophy, it is unclear whether normoglycemia will be an effective treatment for these conditions.[34]

The most metabolically reliable way to establish near-normoglycemia is a pancreatic transplant. There are several different types of transplants available, with or without a kidney transplant or islet cell transplants. Patients receiving transplants often have had diabetes for a long time and have established DPN. The results have reflected this, with only modest improvements. It also took more than three years to see improvement while the neuropathy stabilized.[14]

ARIs respond to the ability of glucose to increase the polyol pathway. The goal of therapy is to decrease the intracellular level of sorbitol in the nerve.[32] The only ARI currently in clinical practice is epalrestat, which is only used in Japan. The result of the studies were summarized by Boulton as "too small, too few, too short, and too late." The ARIs were unable to inhibit sorbitol accumulation; there were not enough subjects in the studies; the trials occurred for a limited time; and DPN was usually well established by the time the ARIs were given. Several of the ARIs were withdrawn because of toxicity.[7]

Other pathogenic treatments include antioxidants, growth factors, and IVIG. Some examples of antioxidants include vitamin E, vitamin C, and a-lipoic acid. Antioxidants are supposed to decrease oxygen free radicals. Some studies cite equivocal results and others note some improvement.[21] NGF is supposed to increase nerve regeneration and establish nerve growth. Studies have been ineffective.[1] IVIG therapy was studied in 21 patients and showed favorable results. IVIG is generally well tolerated and safe. On rare occasions it can result in an anaphylactic reaction. Autoimmune-mediated pathogenesis is a small percentage of DPN so IVIG can be used only for a small percentage of patients.[32] Other treatments mentioned include C-peptide, protein kinase C, and vasodilators. It is worth noting that the main treatment that has been shown to work is normoglycemia. The second most used treatment, ARIs, is used only in Japan.

Symptomatic Treatment

Symptomatic treatment of the pain in DPN is probably one of the most important roles of a physiatrist. It is a difficult management issue because there is a multitude of pain syndromes associated with DPN. Pathology of pain can originate from the nerve terminals, the axon, abnormal activation of the spinal cord synapses or peripheral sympathetic neurons, or abnormalities in the central pain regions of the brain. There is no single correct way to treat DPN pain. Often it requires patience and trial-and-error to develop an effective regimen.[32] The first step in therapy is to exclude nondiabetic causes. Some examples include malignant disease, toxins such as alcohol, infection, medication such as chemotherapeutics, and metabolic causes. Education, support, and practical measures such as using a bed cradle to lift sheets off the skin are the next step. Finally, it is important to stabilize glycemic control.[7]

When changing glycemic regimens, it is worth noting the syndrome of acute painful neuropathy. This syndrome is characterized by acute onset, severe pain, pain in the legs (worse at night), weight loss, and poor control of hyperglycemia. Patients often have a near normal neurologic examination. Acute painful neuropathy can be precipitated by an improvement in glycemic control. Medications do not normally help this condition. It can take 6 to 18 months for the symptoms to resolve.[32]

The next step is pharmacologic treatment. Boulton and colleagues[4] suggest the sequence of tricyclic antidepressants (TCAs) to anticonvulsants to opioid or opioid-like drugs to a pain clinic referral. All anticonvulsants seem to have the same efficacy in randomized controlled studies. Specific pain patterns do seem to respond more to specific combinations of medications.

Paresthesias, dysesthesias, and lancinating pain occur because of diabetic-related changes to unmyelinated C fibers. These fibers use substance P as a neurotransmitter. Type C pain is helped by TCAs, especially combined with fluphenazine. The side effects of TCAs include drowsiness, lethargy, fatigue, dry mouth, blurred vision, urinary retention, and orthostasis. Fluphenazine can cause shakiness. Anticonvulsants such as phenytoin, carbamazepine, and gabapentin could also help this type of pain.

Superficial burning and allodynia can be helped with capsaicin cream or isosorbide dinitrate spray. Capsaicin cream needs to be used carefully in sensitive areas. Anticonvulsants can also help focal neuropathies or pain from mononeuropathies. Anticonvulsants such as gabapentin and carbamazepine can cause dizziness, nausea, rash, marrow toxicity, and leukopenia. A-fiber pain is often a deep-seated, gnawing, dull pain that is most effectively helped with tramadol, dextromethorphan, or antidepressants.[3,14]

One of the main challenges in the treatment of diabetic pain is choosing the right medication. One tool is known as the Numbers Needed to Treat (NNT). The NNT documents the number of patients needed to be treated before one patient achieves 50% pain relief. For TCAs, NNT is 1.4, for dextromethorphan 1.9, for carbamazepine 3.3, for tramadol 3.4, for gabapentin 3.7, for capsaicin 5.9, for selective serotonin-reuptake inhibitors (SSRIs) 6.7, and for mexiletine 10.[14] This comparison can be helpful in developing a treatment plan focused on the patient's individual needs and responses to medication.

TCA medications have been shown to be efficacious and are still used as first-line agents in many centers. TCAs have the advantage of being inexpensive and their side effect profiles are well known. These medications work by inhibiting the reuptake of norepinephrine and serotonin at synapses of central pain nerves in the brain, and seem to move beyond the role of antidepressant. TCAs have been shown to relieve pain equally in patients with and without depression. Amitriptyline and imipramine are the best studied of the TCAs. The dose starts at 25 mg before bed and can be gradually increased to a maximum dose of 150 mg; this is done to avoid the fatigue and lethargy that commonly occur with TCAs. Anticholinergic effects are often limiting; they include dry mouth, arrhythmias, glaucoma, and urinary retention, especially in elderly patients. Desipramine may be better tolerated than amitriptyline. Sometimes in severe cases combination therapy is more effective than monotherapy, for example, combining TCAs with tranquilizers or even transcutaneous electrotherapy.[4,7]

SSRIs include paroxetine, fluoxetine, and citalopram. SSRIs inhibit presynaptic uptake of serotonin. Paroxetine is more efficacious than fluoxetine. Citalopram was shown to be efficacious at 40 mg/day. SSRIs rarely cause troublesome side effects, but may increase the risk of upper gastrointestinal bleeds.

Anticonvulsants have a long history of use with neuropathic pain. Gabapentin is the most commonly prescribed anticonvulsant, being efficacious for DPN-related pain. Gabapentin can be started at 300 mg at night and gradually titrated to therapeutic range (1.8 g/d) based on symptomatic response. Pregabalin is related structurally to gabapentin, and has the advantage of being given twice a day versus three divided doses in the case of gabapentin.[4] Gabapentin's main side effects include dizziness, somnolence, headache, and diarrhea. Carbamazepine is also efficacious in clinical trials. Like the other anticonvulsants, it should be started low at 100 mg twice a day and gradually increased for symptoms. Laboratory work is required every three months to monitor for leukopenia.[32] Phenytoin is sometimes used, though its efficacy has not been shown. Phenytoin can cause a hyperosmolar diabetic coma. Topiramate, another anticonvulsant, can lower blood pressure, improve lipid profiles, and decrease insulin resistance.[14]

Analgesics are generally not shown to be efficacious. Narcotics are discouraged because of constipation and possible addiction. Nonsteroidal anti-inflammatory drugs and tramadol have been shown to work in some cases. Tramadol has similar side effects to opioids. Topical treatments such as capsaicin and topical nitrates can be effective. Capsaicin is most useful for localized treatment. Studies on capsaicin have been short term. Topical nitrate can relieve overall pain and burning in DPN. Physical therapies are useful at any phase of treatment. Transcutaneous electrostimulation has probably been studied the most. Acupuncture has been shown to be helpful in unmasked studies.[7,14]

SUMMARY

DPN is a common disorder that can lead to limb loss and death. Up to 50% of DPN patients can be asymptomatic. Many of the symptoms of DPN contribute to the cascade that leads to limb loss. Symptoms include pain, weakness, unsteadiness, ataxia, and falls. Some of the most prominent changes occur to sensation. The degree of heterogeneity in the clinical manifestations of DPN makes diagnosing this condition difficult. Diagnostic studies such as direct biopsy, skin punch biopsy, and QST are reviewed in this article. Electrophysiologic studies can pinpoint distribution and narrow the differential diagnosis. EMG and NCS help determine distribution; they differentiate focal from multifocal problems, define symmetry, identify proximal from distal, and demonstrate motor and sensory involvement. NCS can specify the segment of the nerve involved. The tests can also distinguish acute from chronic changes and whether a neuropathy is length dependent. All these factors can help rule out conditions not related to diabetes and define the type of neuropathy involved. This article reviews several different classification systems, focusing on Thomas' modified system with rapidly reversible hyperglycemia, generalized symmetric polyneuropathies, and focal and multifocal neuropathies. The pathogenesis of DPN is multifactorial with the main categories being metabolic and ischemic. Treatment falls into two categories, those affecting pathogenesis such as glycemic control and ARIs, and those providing symptomatic treatment such as antidepressants and anticonvulsants. This article reviews the characteristics, diagnosis, electrodiagnosis, classification, pathogenesis, and treatment of DPN.

REFERENCES

1. Greene DA, Stevens MJ, Feldman EL. Diabetic neuropathy: scope of the syndrome. Am J Med 1999;107(2):2–8.
2. Arezzo JCA. New developments in the diagnosis of diabetic neuropathy. Am J Med 1999;107(2):9–16.
3. Vinik A, Mehrabyan A. Diabetic neuropathies. Med Clin North Am 2004;88(4): 947–99.
4. Boulton AJ, Vinik AI, Arezzo JC, et al. Diabetic neuropathies: a statement by the American Diabetes Association. Diabetes Care 2005;28(4):956–62.
5. Apfel SC. Introduction to diabetic neuropathy. Am J Med 1999;107(2):1.
6. Llewelyn JG. The diabetic neuropathies: types, diagnosis and management. J Neurol Neurosurg Psychiatry 2003;74(90002):ii15–9.
7. Boulton AJ, Malik RA, Arezzo JC, et al. Diabetic somatic neuropathies. Diabetes Care 2004;27(6):1458–86.
8. Cohen JA, Jeffers BW, Faldut D, et al. Risks for sensorimotor peripheral neuropathy and autonomic neuropathy in non-insulin-dependent diabetes mellitus (NIDDM). Muscle Nerve 1998;21(1):72–80.

9. Kles KA, Vinik AI. Pathophysiology and treatment of diabetic peripheral neuropathy: the case for diabetic neurovascular function as an essential component. Curr Diabetes Rev 2006;2(2):131–45.

10. Apfel SC, Asbury AK, Bril V, et al. Positive neuropathic sensory symptoms as endpoints in diabetic neuropathy trials. J Neurol Sci 2001;189(1–2):3–5.

11. Perkins BA, Ngo M, Bril V. Symmetry of nerve conduction studies in different stages of diabetic polyneuropathy. Muscle Nerve 2002;25(2):212–7.

12. Thomas PK. Classification, differential diagnosis, and staging of diabetic peripheral neuropathy. Diabetes 1997;46(Suppl 2):S54–7.

13. Sima AA, Thomas PK, Ishii D, et al. Diabetic neuropathies. Diabetologia 1997; 40(Suppl 3):B74–7.

14. Bansal V, Kalita J, Misra UK. Diabetic neuropathy. Postgrad Med J 2006;82(964): 95–100.

15. England JD, Gronseth GS, Franklin G, et al. Evaluation of distal symmetric polyneuropathy: the role of autonomic testing, nerve biopsy, and skin biopsy (an evidence-based review). Muscle Nerve 2009;39(1):106–15.

16. Shy ME, Frohman EM, So YT, et al. Quantitative sensory testing: report of the therapeutics and technology assessment Subcommittee of the American Academy of Neurology. Neurology 2003;60(6):898–904.

17. Perkins BA, Bril V. Diabetic neuropathy: a review emphasizing diagnostic methods. Clin Neurophysiol 2003;114(7):1167–75.

18. England JD, Gronseth GS, Franklin G, et al. Distal symmetric polyneuropathy: a definition for clinical research: report of the American Academy of Neurology, the American Association of Electrodiagnostic Medicine, and the American Academy of Physical Medicine and Rehabilitation. Neurology 2005;64(2): 199–207.

19. Arezzo JC. The use of electrophysiology for the assessment of diabetic neuropathy. Neurosci Res Commun 1997;21(1):13–23.

20. Albers JW. Clinical neurophysiology of generalized polyneuropathy. J Clin Neurophysiol 1993;10(2):149–66.

21. Dyck P. Diabetic neuropathy. 2nd edition. Philadelphia: W.B. Saunders; 1999.

22. Dumitru D. Electrodiagnostic medicine. 2nd edition. Philadelphia: Hanley & Belfus; 2002.

23. Arezzo JC, Zotova E. Electrophysiologic measures of diabetic neuropathy: mechanism and meaning. Int Rev Neurobiol 2002;50:229–55.

24. Donofrio PD, Albers JW. AAEM minimonograph #34: polyneuropathy: classification by nerve conduction studies and electromyography. Muscle Nerve 1990; 13(10):889–903.

25. Hendriksen PH, Oey PL, Wieneke GH, et al. Subclinical diabetic neuropathy: similarities between electrophysiological results of patients with Type 1 (insulin-dependent) and Type 2 (non-insulin-dependent) diabetes mellitus. Diabetologia 1992;35(7):690–5.

26. Watkins PJ. Diabetic autonomic neuropathy. N Engl J Med 1990;322(15):1078–9.

27. Jackson CE, Barohn RJ. Diabetic neuropathic cachexia: report of a recurrent case. J Neurol Neurosurg Psychiatry 1998;64(6):785–7.

28. Godil A, Berriman D, Knapik S, et al. Diabetic neuropathic cachexia. West J Med 1996;165(6):382–5.

29. Ross MA. Neuropathies associated with diabetes. Med Clin North Am 1993;77(1): 111–24.

30. Bays HE, Pfeifer MA. Peripheral diabetic neuropathy. Med Clin North Am 1988; 72(6):1439–64.

31. Tomlinson D, Gardiner N. Diabetic neuropathies: components of etiology. J Peripher Nerv Syst 2008;13(2):112–21.
32. Vinik AI. Diabetic neuropathy: pathogenesis and therapy. Am J Med 1999; 107(2B):17S–26S.
33. Ward JD. The diabetic leg. Diabetologia 1982;22(3):141–7.
34. Parry GJ. Management of diabetic neuropathy. Am J Med 1999;107(2):27–33.
35. The effect of intensive diabetes therapy on the development and progression of neuropathy. The Diabetes Control and Complications Trial Research Group. Ann Intern Med 1995;122(8):561–8.

Pre-Operative Rehabilitation Evaluation of the Dysvascular Patient Prior to Amputation

Kevin N. Hakimi, MD[a,b,*]

KEYWORDS

- Amputation • Rehabilitation • Diabetes mellitus
- Diabetes complications • Peripheral vascular diseases

The relationship between dysvascular diseases, specifically diabetes mellitus (DM) and peripheral vascular disease (PVD), and amputation risk is well established. Eighty-two percent of all amputations in the United States are due to dysvascular causes. Ninety-seven percent of these are lower-extremity amputations, including transmetatarsal, transtibial (TTA), and transfemoral amputations (TFA). Since 1980, the population of people living in the United States with DM has more than doubled to a current prevalence of 7.7% overall and 18.4% for those over age 65.[1] As the US population ages and the prevalence of dysvascular diseases increases, the number of older dysvascular amputees also will increase. It is predicted that the number of lower-extremity amputations in the geriatric population will rise from 28,000 per year in 2001 to 58,000 per year by 2030.[2] Trends in level of amputation in the dysvascular population also have been changing over the past few decades, with a stronger emphasis on preserving the knee joint, if possible, to improve the probability of successful prosthetic fitting. In a study of major lower-extremity amputations at a large academic medical center on the East Coast, 73% of performed procedures were TTAs and only 26% were TFAs.[3] There seem to be, however, many regional differences regarding the level of amputation trends. In a population-based study done in Minnesota, which examined all lower-extremity amputations in one county over a 20-year

[a] Department of Rehabilitation Medicine, University of Washington School of Medicine, 1959 NE Pacific Street, Seattle, WA 98159, USA
[b] Rehabilitation Care Services, VA Puget Sound Health Care System, RCS-117, 1660 South Columbian Way, Seattle, WA 98108, USA
* Corresponding author: VA Puget Sound Health Care System, RCS-117, 1660 South Columbian Way, Seattle, WA 98108, USA
E-mail address: khakimi@u.washington.edu

Phys Med Rehabil Clin N Am 20 (2009) 677–688
doi:10.1016/j.pmr.2009.06.015
1047-9651/09/$ – see front matter. Published by Elsevier Inc.

pmr.theclinics.com

period, a 64% TTA rate versus 36% TFA rate was reported. Two other studies reported even lower TTA rates, from 55% to 60%, and TFA rates as 40% to 45%.[4,5]

GENERAL OUTCOMES

Mortality after amputation in dysvascular patients is high. In a retrospective review of 788 patients undergoing major lower-extremity amputation at an academic tertiary center, overall 30-day mortality of 8.6% was reported, but a considerably higher rate of 16.5% was found for those undergoing TFA. At 1 and 5 years after amputation, overall survival of this group was reported at 69.7% and 34.7%, respectively, and again was significantly worse for the TFA population.[3] Similarly, another retrospective chart review of 154 patients at a university hospital and a Department of Veterans Affairs hospital, reported 1- and 3-year survival rates after major lower-extremity amputation as 78% and 55%, respectively.[4] Another study, based solely in the United States veterans population, found a 7-year survival rate of 39%.[5] Conversion rates from TTA to TFA in these studies ranged from 9.4% to 11%. Recent studies have begun to focus on functional outcome for dysvascular patients undergoing amputation. One-year functional prosthetic use rates, ranging from 23% to 77% after major lower-extremity dysvascular amputations, have been reported.[4–7]

MULTIDISCIPLINARY APPROACH

The loss of a limb can have significant functional consequences and may lead to the loss of independence for many older dysvascular patients. Proper rehabilitation evaluation and management is crucial to ensure successful outcomes for these patients. Rehabilitation should be focused on improving function for all these patients, maximizing independence, addressing psychological needs related to limb loss, and ensuring that quality of life is maintained. These goals are crucial for patients who are prescribed prosthetic limbs and for patients who will not be able to ambulate with a prosthetic limb. The approach to dysvascular amputees, as for many other rehabilitation populations, requires a skilled multidisciplinary team that participates in evaluation of patients not only post-operatively but also pre-operatively.

Although traumatic amputations often are performed under emergent situations, which preclude significant pre-operative evaluation from a multidisciplinary care team, patients presenting with diabetic foot infections and critical limb ischemia should have a team evaluation. Although some dysvascular patients present with urgent infections that require immediate surgical intervention, in most cases amputations can be delayed until patients have had appropriate evaluations completed. Delay often is necessary to treat any active infection prior to definitive amputation. Dysvascular patients, therefore, can benefit from the expertise of a multidisciplinary team that can initiate an appropriate amputee-focused rehabilitation plan of care based on a patient's unique biopsychosocial profile. Biologic, functional, social, and psychological factors must be evaluated and discussed with the team, and an appropriate surgical and rehabilitation plan can be developed and discussed with patients prior to amputation.

The members of a preoperative amputation team can vary greatly between institutions depending on the resources available and the organization of the institution (**Fig. 1**). As with all rehabilitation teams, crucial members are physiatrist, physical therapist, occupational therapist, social worker, rehabilitation psychologist, recreation therapist, and vocational counselor. An amputee team additionally needs to include wound care nurse specialists, prosthetists, orthotists, and a surgical team. The members of a surgical team may vary from hospital to hospital but most often include vascular and orthopedic surgeons and podiatrists. Specifically, for

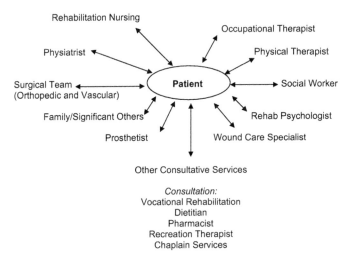

Fig. 1. Example of a typical patient-centered multidisciplinary amputee care team.

dysvascular patients, an evaluation by vascular surgery is crucial to evaluate blood flow with regard to wound healing and to plan any potential revascularization procedures.

Ideally, a team should be involved in the full spectrum of amputation prevention and amputee care once amputation occurs, including foot ulcer prevention, wound care, pre-operative evaluation, surgical care, post-operative care, prosthetic fitting, and lifelong follow-up regarding amputee care. It should be stressed that the role of rehabilitation does not begin post-operatively but must be fully integrated into the continuum of care to ensure quality care and optimal patient outcomes.

The pre-operative process starts with lower-extremity ulcer prevention in patients who are at high risk of foot ulcers related to DM and PVD. Periodic evaluation of sensation and blood flow and identification of biomechanical foot deformities is crucial in prevention of ulcers and eventual amputation. A team working with a primary care provider can help optimize medical status, make appropriate diagnostic referrals, and prescribe appropriate footwear and orthotics.

For patients who develop wounds, evaluation by a wound care specialist to determine the cause of the ulcer and treatment plan is required. Often, to hasten wound healing, non–weight-bearing status is prescribed for patients; in that case, necessary equipment to decrease weight bearing on the affected limb must be prescribed. Patients also may benefit from proper training by a physical therapist to properly use a prescribed assistive device and to demonstrate that they can properly transfer or ambulate without weight bearing on the affected extremity. A team also must take into account the amount of deconditioning that rapidly occurs in this population as a result of limiting weight bearing and prescribe exercise programs that can be accomplished without worsening a foot ulcer. For patients with evidence of ischemia or poorly healing wounds, the involvement of the vascular surgery team is crucial to determine if there are any specific vascular interventions that can be performed to improve blood flow and wound healing. When wounds are not healing and amputation is considered, a physiatrist should evaluate patients (if not already involved in the care of the patients). The prevention of diabetic foot ulcers and the treatment of diabetic infections are discussed in articles by authors, Howard, Miller and Henry, elsewhere in this issue.

Inpatient evaluation of dysvascular patients often revolves around patients with a rapidly worsening infected diabetic ulcer and worsening systemic symptoms or patients with worsening lower-extremity ischemia and rest pain. For these patients, a rapid assessment of the situation is crucial to determining the need for amputation surgery, appropriate level of amputation, pre-operative and post-operative rehabilitation plans, and patient goals. For inpatients and outpatients facing a pending amputation, many factors must be considered in the pre-operative evaluation. Rehabilitation evaluation should not only focus on patients with future prosthetic ambulation potential but also provide treatment of patients for whom ambulation is unlikely. These patients also need rehabilitation interventions to maintain and improve their mobility and activities of daily living (ADL) functions. This article reviews the key factors to evaluate and consider when evaluating dysvascular patients before a potential amputation. The same factors also apply to patients who are evaluated by a rehabilitation team post-operatively.

HISTORY

As in all patient evaluations, accurate, detailed history of patient condition is crucial to developing accurate assessment and recommendations. Key components of patient history as related to potential amputation are discussed later and outlined in **Table 1**.

Table 1
Key history items in preoperative amputee patients

1. Premorbid Functional Status
  a. Mobility
    - Distance ambulated
    - Amount of physical assistance
    - Use of ambulatory aid
    - Factors that limit ambulation (shortness of breath, balance, claudication)
    - Use of manual or power wheelchair
    - History of falls
  b. ADL
    - Assistance needed for basic ADLs (dressing, bathing)
    - Assistance needed for advanced ADLs (cooking, cleaning)
    - Driving status
2. Social history
  a. Social support system
    - Single versus married/partnered/significant other
    - Other available support (children, friends, neighbors, coworkers)
    - Community support/involvement (volunteer activities, church groups)
  b. Home environment
    - Number of stairs to entry and inside
    - Accessibility of house including bathrooms to wheelchair use
  c. Vocational history
    - Past and current vocational status
3. Past medical history
  a. Previous ulcers/amputations
  b. Cardiopulmonary disease (CAD, CHF, COPD, current use of O_2)
  c. PVD disease and claudication symptoms
  d. End-stage complication of diabetes: retinopathy, nephropathy, peripheral neuropathy
  e. Other neurologic condition: stroke, dementia, etc.
  f. Musculoskeletal disorders: lower-extremity osteoarthritis, low back pain
  g. Psychological status: depression, PTSD, anxiety

Premorbid Functional Status

In addition to obtaining the standard parts of patient history, it is crucial to obtain an accurate and complete functional history. It often is easiest to obtain a functional history by asking patients directly and reading chart notes if patients are poor historians. It is not uncommon for patients, however, to be unable to give detailed accurate information due to pain, sedation, dementia, or delirium. Consultants must try to obtain information from other sources, such as patient caregivers and families, in order to get an accurate functional status. Inaccurate understanding of patient functional status can occur and may lead to uninformed recommendations regarding appropriate level of amputation. For example, patients with mild dementia and a history of hemiparesis secondary to stroke may grossly overestimate their mobility even though they have been a primary wheelchair user for years. Conversely, some patients who are admitted in a wheelchair are labeled as nonambulatory when they may be walking for significant parts of the day and for whom the ability to maintain ambulation (eg, into their bathroom) may be crucial to maintaining independence. Two studies addressing ambulatory status prior to amputation or revascularization have reported that between 15% and 16% of patients were nonambulators at the time of pre-operative evaluation. In both of the studies, patients who were nonambulatory at the time of presentation had a low likelihood of ambulating after amputation.[4,7,8]

Often, functional status at the time patients are admitted to a hospital does not reflect true functional history. Usually, current functional status is limited by the wound on the residual limb being considered for amputation and possibly by wounds on the contralateral limb. Patients may have been placed on non–weight-bearing status for a few days or possibly many months in an attempt to achieve wound healing. The longer patients have been nonambulatory, the more difficult it may be to achieve successful prosthetic ambulation. Prolonged wheelchair use leading to muscle weakness, cardiopulmonary deconditioning, and contracture development influences the pre-operative rehabilitation assessment.

Functional status history needs to be detailed and must include not only the amount of ambulation occurring but also the setting and context of ambulation, such as community versus household ambulation. For example, patients may first report they can walk five blocks but when questioned further, they may report that they have not actually done this in over a year. Other factors to document include the ability to walk on uneven surfaces, ability to use stairs, use of assistive devices, and fall history. ADL history (cooking, bathing, toilet transfers, dressing, and so forth) also must be fully investigated. With regards to mobility and ADL function, the amount of assistance needed from a caregiver or relative for each activity must be explored. Patients who already are homebound but ambulatory prior to amputation are at higher risk of not wearing a prosthetic and not being able to maintain independent living status after amputation.[7] Again, identifying these patients who have a marginal functional status prior to amputation can help guide an amputation team with regards to appropriate surgical care and instituting a pre-operative rehabilitation program.

Cognition and Psychological History

The cognitive status of patients is paramount in assessing their future success with prosthesis. Significant dementia may preclude prosthetic use in patients who otherwise physically are candidates. Poor cognition may interfere with the ability to safely don and doff a prosthesis or to properly evaluate a residual and contralateral limb for ulceration. Similar to functional history, patient baseline cognitive status is not always apparent at the time of evaluation. In the setting of impending amputation, many factors may cause temporary changes in cognitive status, especially in those patients with baseline mild dementia. Acute infection, pain medications, depression, uremia, sedation, and sundowning all may worsen patients' cognitive status. In these situations, consultants must obtain information from hospital staff, caregivers, and family to fully understand patients' true cognitive abilities. A speech pathology consultation to further evaluate the cognitive abilities of patients can provide crucial data to a rehabilitation team. Dementia is associated with a low probability of future prosthetic use and a low probability of maintaining independent living after amputation.[6,7] In one study, low scores on a 15-word test of short-term memory and delayed recall at 2 weeks after amputation in vascular patients predicted poor functional outcome.[6] More recently, another study showed that mobility and number of hours of prosthetic use at 6 months after lower-extremity amputation was significantly less for patients with deficits in memory and executive functioning.[9]

The mental health of prospective amputees also must be evaluated. Psychological comorbidities, such as depression, anxiety, posttraumatic stress disorder, and substance abuse, may play a role not only in unsuccessful prosthetic fitting but also in preventing the achievement of an overall satisfactory quality of life. A consultant must obtain a detailed psychological history regarding the course of symptoms, types of treatment, and current status of the mental illness. Amputation itself can be associated with depression even without a history of depression premorbidly. The involvement of a mental health provider prior to amputation should always be strongly considered even in those without premorbid psychological history to help with adjustment to limb loss.

Vision

Visual deficits are common in the dysvascular patient population, particularly in patients with DM who develop diabetic retinopathy. The development of diabetic retinopathy is predicted to increase significantly over the next 50 years as the population ages and as the prevalence of diabetes increases.[10] Poor vision can affect successful prosthetic ambulation. Sufficient vision is needed to properly don a prosthetic limb and to ensure the suspension system is engaged properly. Vision also is essential to ensure monitoring of a residual limb and contralateral limb for ulceration development. Once ambulating, vision is important from a safety perspective for avoiding objects and being able to see uneven terrain or obstacles ahead. Poor vision does not necessarily preclude prosthetic use but it most likely limits it and requires more social support and a more detailed rehabilitation plan of care to achieve success. There are various methods of altering prosthesis components to provide needed tactile cues to properly don a prosthetic. Patients with poor vision also may benefit from referral to blindness rehabilitation specialists to improve their functional outcome.

Cardiopulmonary Status and Obesity

Ambulating with a prosthetic limb at a given speed requires significantly more energy expenditure than for able-bodied individuals. Most geriatric amputees compensate for this increased energy demand by decreasing their self-selected walking speed. For any given distance walked, however, the efficiency of ambulation is decreased for this population. The amount of increased energy expenditure depends on the level of amputation and on whether or not patients are bilateral or unilateral amputees. In younger patients with traumatic amputation, increased metabolic demands associated with prosthetic ambulation are usually not a significant barrier to success. In the dysvascular population, cardiopulmonary status must be evaluated carefully to determine how it will effect ambulation or to determine whether or not ambulation is precluded. For unilateral vascular TTA, metabolic cost is estimated to increase by 40%, and for unilateral TFA, metabolic cost increases by 100%.[11]

The higher prevalence of coexistent coronary heart disease (CHD) in the dysvascular patient population also affects patients' future outcome. Patients with diabetes have a higher prevalence of CHD, have a greater extent of myocardial ischemia, and are more likely to have a myocardial infarction. Besides known CHD, patients may have other cardiopulmonary limitations, such as congestive heart failure (CHF) or chronic obstructive pulmonary disease (COPD), which may limit their exercise capacity. If at the time of pre-operative evaluation, patients already have CHD, CHF, or COPD, severely limiting their function, a poor prognosis for prosthetic ambulation or even successful manual wheelchair propulsion may be predicted. Some studies have shown the presence of advanced CHD to be a statistically significant factor associated with not wearing a prosthetic.[7] Most patients who have limited cardiopulmonary status, however, still should be considered for and prescribed prosthesis. Again, most of these patients can compensate for their suboptimal cardiopulmonary status by decreasing their self-selected walking speed. This may prelude practical use of a prosthetic for community ambulation but may allow use of a prosthetic device in the home environment. For these individuals, it is crucial to make sure that their cardiopulmonary diseases are managed optimally and that they maintain a cardiovascular fitness program in the pre-operative, perioperative, and postoperative period. Enrollment of patients in cardiac rehabilitation programs also should be considered in order to improve cardiopulomonary status and to improve the ability to ambulate with a prosthesis post amputation. Patients who are on bed rest in the hospital go through a rapid deconditioning process. All older dysvascular amputees, regardless of their cardiopulmonary history, should be instructed in ways to maintain cardiopulmonary fitness in order to avoid the effects of deconditioning.

Obesity is a growing epidemic in the United States with more than 66% of the population overweight (body mass index >25) and 31% of the population obese (body mass index >30).[12] Obesity is associated with many risk factors and is thought to be a barrier to ambulation with a prosthetic. Although actual prosthetic fit may be more difficult and may require specialized components, there is evidence in the literature that suggests obesity does not seem to effect prosthetic usage, maintenance of ambulation, overall survival, or independent living status.[13]

End-stage Renal Disease

The presence of end-stage renal disease (ESRD) also is associated with significantly poorer outcome in dysvascular amputee patients compared with those patients with normal kidney function. Five-year survival in patients with renal failure and major lower-extremity amputation was found to be only 14.4% compared with 42.4% in those without renal failure.[2] ESRD also was associated with not wearing a prosthesis and with failure of ambulation. Patients with ESRD can be successful ambulators but the process is more difficult secondary to their comorbid medical conditions. Patients on chronic dialysis who entered a rehabilitation program after major lower-extremity amputation had longer hospitalizations but similar outcomes compared to the nonuremic patients.[14]

Age

Although age itself should not be used as a single factor to predict success ambulating with a prosthesis, increased age is associated with poorer outcome and a higher likelihood of losing independent living status. For elderly patients, it is crucial to fully evaluate all other pertinent factors, paying particular attention to social support of patients and the other medical comorbidities. Patients over 70 years old had a 3 times higher likelihood of not wearing a prosthesis and 4 times greater chance of losing functional independence 1 year after amputation.[7]

Social Support and Home Environment

The home environment and social support of patients must be explored so that appropriate rehabilitation planning can begin. The need for early rehabilitation after an amputation may be influenced by the lack of social support or major architectural barriers of the home. Some patients after surgery are able to return home with support and proper equipment while they are awaiting wound healing and prosthetic fitting. Other patients may require subacute or nursing home level of care for wound healing and rehabilitation. A pre-operative consultant should begin discussing various disposition options prior to surgery so that patients and family members can start making appropriate plans. Assistance of a social worker should also be requested for patients for whom disposition may be difficult. For some patients, based on the level of amputation performed, returning to their current home may not be an option. For elderly vascular patients who live in a second-floor apartment without an elevator, TTA gives patients a better opportunity of remaining independent compared to TFA. These factors must be considered pre-operatively and discussed with the operative team prior to surgery.

Status of the Contralateral Limb

Preoperative evaluation of patients for amputation not only includes the threatened limb but also must include the contralateral limb. In the case of dysvascular patients, the contralateral limb is inherently at high risk of future amputation, which further threatens patients' functional status. Current ulcers or the development of new ulcers affects the ability of patients to become a successful ambulator after amputation. As an amputee, the intact limb experiences greater mechanical forces and is at an even higher risk for possible ulceration. Careful physical examination and prescription of appropriate footwear and or orthotic must be considered in the contralateral limb.

In many cases, the contralateral limb already may have an amputation. For patients who already have a lower-extremity amputation related to diabetes or vascular disease, the risk of future contralateral or ipsilateral major reamputation (Syme's amputation, TTA, or TFA) is high. In a study of 277 diabetic patients, those who underwent an initial unilateral amputation had a contralateral major limb amputation rate at 1 year, 3 years, and 5 years of 11.6%, 44.1%, and 53.3%, respectively.[15] For those who are already long-term nonambulators, the amputation of the contralateral limb may have less bearing on ambulatory status; however, it affects overall mobility. For example, patients may be dependant on the remaining limb for transfers. If an amputation occurs, a transfer limb is a consideration; therefore, discussion of the advantages of a below-knee amputation are communicated with the surgical team. In patients who currently are ambulatory, the significantly increased energy expenditure requirement needed to ambulate with bilateral prostheses must be considered. Patients who are ambulating well with a unilateral prosthesis have the potential to continue doing so as a bilateral amputee. One study that followed patients with dysvascular bilateral TTAs for an average of 4 years after discharge from an inpatient rehabilitation unit after prosthetic fitting found 85% of the surviving patients still wearing their prostheses and walking.[16] The combination of a TTA and TFA in this population most likely has a poorer outcome. Another study of patients with a TTA and contralateral TFA secondary to PVD, found that at an average of 2.99 years from the second amputation, the mortality rate for this population was 68% and an overall poor level of function.[17]

PHYSICAL EXAMINATION

Current physical status of patients must be evaluated to determine whether or not patients have the physical capacity to eventually ambulate with a prosthetic. In addition to a general physical examination, a rehabilitation consultant must focus on certain key areas, including musculoskeletal, neurologic, and cardiopulmonary examination as well as a functional evaluation (**Table 2**).

Musculoskeletal examination should include strength testing not only of the affected limb but also of the contralateral limb and upper extremity limbs. Certain muscles, such as hip flexors, extensors, abductors, and knee extensors and flexors, play crucial roles in prosthetic walking. The importance of maintaining strength in the proximal lower-extremity musculature increases significantly if patients require a TFA versus a TTA due to the need to be able to safely control a prosthetic knee during the gait cycle. Ambulation in the preprosthetic phase requires sole use of the contralateral limb and upper-extremity strength to assist with transfers and ambulation with a walker, crutches, or other assistive devices. Strength deficits may be related to deconditioning or may be related to other disease processes, such as diabetic neuropathy or residuals from a previous cerebrovascular accident. In addition to strength testing, manual dexterity and coordination, especially in the upper extremities, should be evaluated as this can affect ability to don and doff a prosthesis.

Another key element of a physical examination in this population is evaluation of joint range of motion (ROM). ROM should be evaluated carefully and measured with a goniometer in the affected and contralateral limbs. Significant pain or laxity in any joint should be noted. Identification of hip and knee flexion contractures should be noted as they make prosthetic fitting more difficult and require a greater metabolic demand from an amputee during ambulation. The presence of contracture also indicates to an examiner that a patient may have been nonambulatory for a long period

---

Table 2
Key physical examination components in preoperative amputee patients

1. Neurologic
   a. Cognitive evaluation
   b. Cranial nerve examination
   c. Evidence of upper/lower motor neuron lesions
   d. Assessment of peripheral neuropathy
2. Musculoskeletal
   a. Condition of the contralateral limb
   b. Muscle strength (upper and lower extremity)
   c. ROM (upper and lower extremity joints)
   d. Evaluation for joint laxity/instability on key lower-extremity joints
3. Cardiovascular system
   a. Carotid bruits
   b. Peripheral pulses in the lower extremities
   c. Signs of CHF
   d. Peripheral edema
4. Functional evaluation
   a. Bed mobility
   b. Sitting and standing balance (one legged)
   c. Ambulation
   d. Dynamic balance and stability
   e. Motor coordination
   f. Presence of cardiovascular limitations during functional activities

of time. For patients starting to develop contractures due to being nonambulatory, the importance of stretching must be explained. A physical therapy program should be instituted immediately to try to maintain and improve ROM. For patients with severe fixed contractures, prosthetic fitting and ambulation may not be possible. Knee flexion contractures greater than 25° are consistent with difficult fitting and poor outcome related to ambulation.[18]

Balance remains one of the key physical indicators and seems correlated with successful ambulation in amputees. Testing patient balance pre-operatively gives a consultant insight regarding successful ambulation with a prosthesis. Very poor balance pre-operatively indicates that prosthetic ambulation will be more difficult. The most common method of testing balance in this population is the one-legged balance test. A consultant can ask patients to stand on the contralateral leg to see if they are able to balance without assistance. One-legged standing balance at 2 weeks' post amputation is associated with improved ambulatory status at 1 year.[7] In a review analyzing 48 various studies of multiple physical factors affecting walking ability in patients with lower-extremity amputation, only balance had a strong relationship to walking ability.[19] Poor balance can be related to deconditioning and neurologic deficits, such as peripheral neuropathy commonly associated with diabetes or may be related to the normal aging process.

Thorough physical examination of the contralateral extremity needs to be completed. As stated previously, future probability of contralateral amputation is high. The contralateral limb should be evaluated for any skin ulcers, foot deformities, ischemic changes, sensation, and ankle plantar flexion contractures. Appropriate footwear recommendation should be initiated based on physical examination findings.

Functional examination of patients may reveal the most important information regarding future prosthetic function. Patients should demonstrate their bed mobility, transfer, and ambulatory skill to the examiner. Formal evaluation by a physical therapist and occupational therapist can be useful to further test and document current functional status. Examiners must realize that current functional status may be affected by pain, delirium, pain medication, depression, and so forth.

PATIENT EDUCATION

Another key function of rehabilitation consultation is beginning the patient education process regarding life after amputation. Potential limb loss in patients represents a major life event that not only changes physical function but also causes significant psychological distress. Often patients have had no experience interacting with other amputees; therefore, they cannot conceptualize their future function or quality of life after amputation. Many patients have concerns related to their ability to walk, ability to engage in vocational activities, dependency on pain medication, loss of social functioning, and sexual functioning.[20] Although a surgical team is more suited to discussing what happens at the time of surgery, a rehabilitation team is better suited to discussing with patients what happens after surgery. With education, much of the fear and anxiety related to the amputation may be allayed.

The amount of important information that could be shared with potential amputees during the pre-operative period is immense and could potentially overwhelm patients. Information should not be given all during one visit but should be spread out over multiple visits if possible. Education should come from all members of a team, not only a physician. Overall, amputee patients have reported dissatisfaction with the amount of education and information, especially regarding functional outcome.[21] For patients who are having significant trouble adjusting to the concept of amputation, referral to a mental health provider, preferably a rehabilitation psychologist with training in limb loss, should be considered.

On completion of a detailed history and examination and collaboration with a surgical team, some key information should be conveyed to all patients. First, explain the post-operative amputee process as it occurs in the relevant institution. Discussion should include post-operative dressings, participation in physical therapy and occupational therapy post-operatively, potential preprosthetic rehabilitation process, pain (including phantom pain), wound healing time, and the prosthetic fitting process. Based on the information gathered, a consultant should discuss with patients future potential function with and without a prosthesis and the effect the amputation may have on their current living status. It is important for a consultant to inquire about patients' goals and refine the goals based on the clinical scenario. Butler et al. stress the importance for a consultant to be "positively realistic" and to support patient goals but it also is important not to approach patients with false optimism.[20] The amount of information discussed at any visit can be directed by patients. Ask patients what they want to know and what their concerns are regarding amputation. If patients are unsure, writing down questions as they arise and having a member of the team return later is useful. There also are various patient education materials for patients who undergo amputation. The Amputee Coalition of America (www.amputee-coalition. org) is a good resource for these materials.

The use of peer support in the pre-operative period also can be helpful for answering patients' questions and allaying fears. Peer support can encompass the formation of a peer support group or use of a peer visitation program in which individuals who already have had an amputation can visit with patients pre- or post-operatively. Seeing another amputee who has gone through a rehabilitation process can be helpful in the overall educational process and may help patients cope from a psychological perspective. Many hospitals have peer visitation networks and the Amputee Coalition of America maintains a group of trained volunteers from which patients can request visits.

SUMMARY

Lower-extremity amputation in the dysvascular population will continue to be a major problem in the US health care system as prevalence rates of diabetes continues to increase. This population of older amputees can have a good functional outcome. Dysvascular patients who are facing impending amputation must be evaluated by a multidisciplinary team that includes a rehabilitative specialist, who should have the expertise to evaluate functional and other factors that affect final outcomes for patients. Rehabilitation evaluation should guide surgical planning and patient education. Specialists also must recognize the psychological effects related to limb loss and initiate appropriate treatment and peer support. This approach helps ensure the best outcome for all patients undergoing amputation regardless of future ambulatory potential.

ACKNOWLEDGMENTS

The author thanks Elizabeth Broussard, MD, for assistance in editing.

REFERENCES

1. American Diabetes Association. Diabetes statistics. Available at: http://www. diabetes.org/diabetes-statistics.jsp. Accessed April 20, 2009.

2. Fletcher D, Andrews K, Hallet J, et al. Trends in rehabilitation after amputation for geriatric patients with vascular disease: implications for future health care resource allocation. Arch Phys Med Rehabil 2002;83:1389–93.

3. Aulivola B, Hile C, Hamdan A, et al. Major lower extremity amputation: outcome of a modern series. Arch Surg 2004;139:395–9.

4. Nehler M, Coll J, Hiatt W, et al. Functional outcome in a contemporary series of major lower extremity amputations. J Vasc Surg 2002;38:7–14.

5. Cruz C, Eidt J, Capps C, et al. Major lower extremity amputations at a Veterans Affairs hospital. Am J Surg 2003;186:449–54.

6. Fletcher D, Andrews L, Butters M, et al. Rehabilitation of the geriatric vascular amputee patient: a population-based study. Arch Phys Med Rehabil 2001;82:776–9.

7. Schoppen T, Boonstra A, Groothoff J, et al. Physical, mental and social predictors of functional outcome in unilateral lower limb amputees. Arch Phys Med Rehabil 2003;84:803–11.

8. Taylor S, Kalbaugh C, Blackhurst D, et al. Preoperative clinical factors predict postoperative functional outcomes after major lower limb amputation: an analysis of 553 consecutive patients. J Vasc Surg 2005;42:227–35.

9. Oneil B, Evans J. Memory and executive function predict mobility rehabilitation outcome after lower extremity amputation. Disabil Rehabil 2009;31:1083–91.

10. Saaddine J, Honeycutt A, Narayan K, et al. Projection of Diabetic Retinopathy and other major eye diseases among people with diabetes mellitus: United States, 2005–2050. Arch Ophthalmol 2008;126:1740–7.

11. Czerniecki J. Rehabilitation in limb deficiency. 1. Gait and motion analysis. Arch Phys Med Rehabil 1996;77:S3–8.

12. American Heart Association. Heart disease and stroke statistics—2009 update web page. Available at: http://www.americanheart.org/presenter.jhtml?identifier=1928. Accessed April 20, 2009.

13. Kalbaugh C, Taylor S, Kalbaugh B, et al. Does obesity predict functional outcome in the dysvascular amputee? Am Surg 2006;72:707–13.

14. Korzet A, Ori Y, Rathaus M, et al. Lower extremity amputations in chronically dialysed patients: a 10 year study. Isr Med Assoc J 2003;5:501–5.

15. Izumi Y, Lee S, Satterfield K, et al. Risk of reamputation in diabetic patients stratified by limb and level of amputation. Diabetes Care 2006;29:566–70.

16. Mac Neill H, Devlin M, Yudin A. Long term outcomes and survival of patients with bilateral transtibial amputations after rehabilitation. Am J Phys Med Rehabil 2008;87:189–96.

17. Bhangu S, Devlin M, Pauley T. Outcomes of individuals with transfemoral and contralateral transtibial amputation due to dysvascular etiologies. Prosthet Orthot Int 2009;33:33–40.

18. Kapp S, Fergason J. Transtibial amputation: prosthetic management. In: Smith D, Michael J, Bowker J, editors. Atlas of amputations and limb deficiencies: surgical, prosthetic and rehabilitation principles. 3rd edition. Rosemont (IL): American Academy of Orthopedic Surgeons; 2004. p. 503–15.

19. Van Velzen J, Van Bennekon C, Van der Woude L, et al. Physical capacity and walking ability after lower limb amputation: a systemic review. Clin Rehabil 2006;20:999–1016.

20. Butler D, Turkal N, Seidl J. Amputation: preoperative psychological preparation. J Am Board Fam Pract 1992;5:69–73.

21. Watanabe Y, McCluskie P, Hakim E, et al. Lower limb amputee patients' satisfaction with information and rehabilitation. Int J Rehabil Res 1999;22:67–9.

Prosthetic Rehabilitation Issues in the Diabetic and Dysvascular Amputee

Heikki Uustal, MD[a,b]

KEYWORDS

- Amputee • Prosthetic rehabilitation • Lower limb amputation
- Diabetic dysvascular disease • Complications of amputation

POST-OPERATIVE EVALUATION

The history and physical examination remain the most important components of post-operative evaluation. A thorough review of patients' previous activities leading up to the amputation is necessary, but there are key issues that have an impact on the immediate care and future care of patients with lower limb amputation. These key issues include the date when the problem first started, which may have limited patient mobility; the date of hospitalization, which may have severely limited patient activity; all surgeries leading up to and including the amputation, in addition to revisions or complications, which may have occurred post-operatively; names of surgeons involved for contact information to obtain further details as necessary or for future issues if complications should occur; and review of pain issues related to the knee amputation itself in addition to pain prior to and after amputation surgery. Three types of pain are defined: surgical pain related to the operation, phantom sensation with a simple awareness of the absent body part, and, phantom pain, in which there are painful or disturbing feelings arising from a missing body part. Treatments and management of these types of pain are reviewed in detail later. Patients must be reassured that adequate pain control will be provided as part of the post-operative rehabilitation program.

It also is important to review and assess patients' post-operative therapy program and level of mobilization just before and after amputation surgery. It is not unusual for patients to have declined functionally as a result of preceeding complications that led to the amputation. Patients who have been non-ambulatory for more than 6 months have a much higher likelihood of complications, such as hip flexion contracture,

[a] JFK-Johnson Rehabilitation Institute, Department of Physical Medicine and Rehabilitation, Edison, NJ 08820, USA
[b] Department of Rehabilitation Services, St. Peter's University Hospital, 254 Easton Ave, New Brunswick, NJ 08901, USA
E-mail address: suustal@aol.com

deconditioning, and depression. Review of recent medications, laboratory tests, and studies that have been done is prudent to have a full awareness of patients' underlying medical conditions before and after amputation surgery.

Current level of function for mobility and self-care serves as a starting point for a therapy program and helps in establishing short-term and long-term goals for patients. Patients with dysvascular disease and diabetes generally have had some time to think and prepare for the limb loss. The psychological adjustments, however, may still be difficult, because of concerns about return to their previous life and family obligations. It is important to inquire about patients' concerns related to limb loss and future function and performance. An appropriate referral to psychological services is necessary to help manage this issue.

A thorough review of patients' prior level of function and activities is helpful in establishing patients' future goals. Carefully review the activities in the home, out of the home, and in the community. Simple questions—such as, When was the last time a patient walked on two feet unassisted?—are helpful in establishing patients' previous level of mobility function. Inquire what distance they could tolerate walking before they became tired, short of breath, or developed chest pain. If they used assistive devices, clarify the type of device and how long it has been used. It is not unusual for patients to forget or slightly exaggerate their performance before amputation; therefore, collaboration with family members is helpful to ensure that the information is correct.

A standard review of systems should be incorporated into the history, including issues such as cardiac disease, chest pain, shortness of breath, and history of myocardial infarction or cardiac surgery. Review of systems should include issues related to falls before and after amputation, which may have been caused by balance disorder, dizziness, vertigo, or vision loss, and issues related to weight gain or loss, nutritional aspects, depression, and overall quality of life. Details of past medical history can be obtained from charts or from patients and, again, should include issues related to cardiopulmonary disease, renal disease, diabetes, and other major medical disease. Questions related to cognitive function, which may relate to early levels of dementia or impairment, are important to include. A social history helps establish what the home situation was and what the social support network was in the past and will be in the future. Details of home setup, such as stairs to enter and exit the house and any stairs or level changes within the house; access to the bedroom, bathroom, and kitchen areas; and doorways with configurations, should be included.[1–4]

Examination of patients should be thorough and comprehensive (key areas are discussed later). In the review of cranial nerves, vision, oral movements, and swallowing issues should be covered carefully. Cognitive assessment and orientation should be assessed thoroughly for early signs of memory changes or dementia. Cardiopulmonary examination should include careful review of heart, lungs, and peripheral pulses, including carotid, femoral, popliteal, dorsalis pedis, and posterior tibialis pulses. Examination of the upper limb should include manual muscle testing of grip, intrinsic hand muscles, biceps, triceps, deltoid and shoulder depressors (pectoralis and latissimus). These muscles are critical for proper use of an assistive device for ambulation with and without a prosthetic. Sensation and fine motor skills in both hands should be assessed carefully as these are helpful in allowing patients to achieve independence in donning and doffing a prosthetic device. Cerebellar function should be assessed for balance issues.

Examination of the lumbar spine, including range of motion for flexion, extension, lateral bending, and rotation, is important because many lower limb amputees suffer lumbar or sacroiliac pain as a result of the biomechanical changes that occur during gait with or without prosthesis. Examination of the lower limb should include manual muscle testing of hip flexion, extension, abduction and adduction, knee flexion and extension, ankle dorsiflexion and plantarflexion, and inversion and eversion.

Overall assessment of skin integrity includes any open wounds, loss of hair, quality of the toenails, peripheral pulses (discussed above), and sensation in the lower limbs, including light touch, pinprick, and proprioceptive feedback. The remaining foot should be inspected carefully for the areas of pressure, callus, or severe dysvascular disease, as indicated by discoloration and cool temperature. Range of motion, including hip extension, knee extension, ankle dorsiflexion, and plantarflexion in the remaining foot, is important to allow patients to resume proper ambulation. Hip flexion and knee flexion contracture are common in hospitalized patients, particularly in patients with lower limb amputation. These may occur unilaterally on the side of amputation or bilaterally as a result of lack of mobility and ambulation for several weeks or months.

Examination of a residual limb should include careful assessment and documentation of the level of amputation with proper nomenclature and establishment of the bony length of the remaining segment. Quality and quantity of soft tissue coverage over the end of an amputation should be documented. Manual palpation of a residual limb to indicate areas of tenderness or increased sensitivity helps plan for tissue tolerance within the prosthetic device. Assessment of the surgical site for evidence of appropriate healing should be documented carefully. Sensation of a residual limb is helpful to identify areas of potential increased risk once use of a prosthesis is instituted. Description of the overall shape of the residual limb, such as bulbous, cylindric, or cone shaped, should be documented to help monitor shaping of the residual limb. Circumferential measurements of a residual limb—proximal, mid, and distal—should be taken to objectively document volume changes and limb shrinking. Any open wounds that are on a residual limb or remaining foot should be measured carefully for length, width, depth, and any undermining. It is helpful to document the quality of the wound in addition to the description of the depth of the tissues and the quality of the tissues remaining. Wound care management is discussed later.

Assessment of the functional capability of patients at the time of examination is helpful, including independence in bed mobility, transfers, sit-to-stand position on remaining limb, and standing balance on the remaining limb. Many patients are unable to stand immediately post-operatively. Most patients should be able to do this within several days after amputation, however. Overall standing balance and endurance should be assessed as part of the examination. If patients have initiated therapy and some mobility, then ambulating with a walker or crutches, including hopping on the remaining leg, should be assessed for strength, endurance, and safety.

PATIENT EDUCATION

After the history and examination of patients are completed, it is the role of physicians and prosthetic and orthotic teams to educate patients and families regarding the entire program associated with prosthetic fitting and training, including a review of medical findings that are relevant to a prosthetic fitting and training program. An estimate of the time frame of prosthetic fitting and training is helpful to families and patients, because they have no sense of how long this process may take. Explanation and demonstration of prosthetic devices, components, and socket design are helpful once patients are ready to receive this information. Many patients have a preconception or false notion about the cosmesis or function of prosthesis, and these should be explored in detail. Establishment of functional goals and expectations, short term and long term, is done as early as possible. This helps patients make plans for discharge from the hospital and management at home. A thorough explanation of the physical demands and energy cost of prosthetic training is helpful for patients with underlying cardiopulmonary disease. Explanation of limitation of prosthetic use, such as impact on driving, climbing ladders, and ambulation outdoors on uneven terrain, should be reviewed as patients try to understand the overall rehabilitation process.[5,6]

Patients should be educated on monitoring the skin on the residual limb and the remaining foot through the process of pre-prosthetic therapy, prosthetic fitting, and prosthetic training. Patients are their own best advocates to ensure proper healing of the residual limb and to prevent any injury or irritation to the remaining foot. The use of proper footwear, on the prosthesis and the remaining foot, is critical and is reviewed later.

Introduction of the other members of a prosthetic team should start early in the rehabilitation program. Each member has a separate role that should be clearly identified to patients and other team members. The physician directing the rehabilitation program is responsible for thorough evaluation of patients and for providing diagnosis, prognosis, and risk evaluation to patients and the remaining team members. If there are issues related to healing or to pain that have an impact on the therapy program or prosthetic fitting, these should be clearly conveyed to the appropriate individuals. Physicians also supervise other members and ensure proper follow-up and monitoring of the response to the treatment program. Physicians are responsible for generating prescriptions for the appropriate therapy program, prosthetic device, footwear for the remaining limb, and medications to manage pain or depression.

A certified prosthetist is a critical member of a prosthetic team and should be invited to participate in the evaluation process and recommendation for prosthetic design. A prosthetist is an expert on material, components, and design issues of prostheses and there should be open discussion with physicians and therapists on the most appropriate and optimal design for individual patients. A certified prosthetist is responsible for fabricating the prosthetic device, fitting of the device, and follow-up for modifications and adjustments of the prosthetic device. A prosthetist should communicate any issues or concerns with the team and provide feedback and follow-up regarding progress with prosthetic fitting and training.

A physical therapist becomes a team member immediately after surgery to initiate a pre-prosthetic therapy program and should be invited to participate in evaluation of patients and make recommendations for a pre-prosthetic and prosthetic therapy program. A physical therapist should be aware of underlying medical conditions and any risks and potential problems related to the amputation surgery as provided by the physician. Physical therapists should provide feedback to the physician and prosthetist related to a patient's progress in muscle strengthening, range of motion, mobility, and self-care tasks. If there are issues or any discomfort during a physical therapy evaluation and treatments that may impair or impact a prosthetic fitting and training program, they should be conveyed immediately to the appropriate team member.

A certified pedorthist should be included to assist in recommendation and fabrication of appropriate footwear for the remaining limb. A pedorthist should be invited to participate in evaluation and management of patients on a regular basis. A pedorthist fabricates appropriate footwear, which often includes extradepth orthopedic-type shoes with a custom-molded foot orthotic to help protect the remaining foot. A pedorthist can participate in the education process related to monitoring and protecting the remaining foot. Regular follow-up with a pedorthist for replacement and adjustment of the footwear is necessary.

Psychological services often are needed for patients after any level of amputation. There is a cognitive and psychological change that occurs after limb loss similar to the grieving process when a friend or family member is lost. There are issues related to family structure, family unit, and interaction with friends that should be addressed by a licensed psychologist. This service should be offered to all patients and, at minimum, screening should take place. If patients seem to be adjusting well, then only periodic re-evaluation may be necessary by a psychologist.

Significant psychological issues that are present or appear later, however, may have a severe impact on the progress of patients in a rehabilitation program, and this information should be conveyed to the physician and other team members as appropriate.

Patients are key members of the prosthetic rehabilitation team. Patients are expected to cooperate with other team members in providing appropriate information throughout the history and examination. Patients are expected to remain compliant with the treatment and recommendations from each of the team members or to convey information if they are unable to be compliant with the treatment program. Patients should be willing to express concerns regarding pain, psychological issues and depression, or social issues that may impair their ability to participate and cooperate with the treatment program.

PRE-PROSTHETIC THERAPY PROGRAM

A physical therapy program should be instituted almost immediately after amputation surgery. Most patients are able to participate in a therapy program, at least incorporating the upper limbs and remaining limb, shortly after surgery. Strengthening and range of motion of the amputation limb may be delayed a few days because of pain issues or concerns on the part of a surgeon; however, these should be treated or addressed as soon as possible. Strengthening of critical muscles to prepare for ambulation with or without a prosthesis is one of the primary goals of a pre-prosthetic program. In the upper limbs, the critical muscles include grip, intrinsic muscles of the hand, elbow extensors, and shoulder depressors. Patients can start a simple program of wheelchair press-ups to help strengthen all these muscles simultaneously. In the lower limb, the critical muscles include hip extensors and abductors, knee extensors, and ankle dorsiflexors and plantarflexors in the remaining limb. It is important to maintain or improve range of motion at the critical joints, specifically hip extension, knee extension, and ankle dorsiflexion and plantarflexion, during the pre-prosthetic time. It is common for patients to lose range of motion at the hip and knee quickly; therefore, full extension of the knee and at least 20° of extension of the hip should be goals during the pre-prosthetic time.

A physical therapist should be involved in shaping and shrinking of the residual limb. It is ideal to have the surgeon wrap a compressive dressing on the residual limb in the operating room immediately after surgery. This may stay on for 1 to 3 days based on surgeon recommendation. Once initial surgical dressing is removed, continued shrinking and shaping of a residual limb occurs with figure-of-eight Ace wrapping of the residual limb 23 hours per day. This Ace wrapping should be rewrapped several times per day to monitor the skin, provide hygiene to the skin, and assess the shape of the residual limb. Patients and families should be educated on proper Ace-wrapping technique. Patients and families, in addition to the medical team, can monitor skin integrity and healing.

Application of a rigid dressing at the time of surgery is an alternative method of management. The rigid plaster or fiberglass dressing prevents the usual post-operative edema from occurring and typically remains in place for 7 to 10 days. Removal of the rigid dressing after 7 days allows for inspection of the skin and surgical site. If there are no complications or concerns, a second rigid dressing can be applied for an additional 7 to 10 days or until the sutures/staples are removed. If patients have increasing pain or fever while the rigid dressing is in place, then the dressing is removed briefly for inspection and reapplied if there are no problems. If there are concerns about healing, then traditional management with Ace wrapping can be instituted at that time.[7,8]

After staples and sutures are removed, shrinker socks can be used for continued shrinking and shaping. Desensitization of a residual limb through tapping, rubbing, or massage can be instituted shortly after amputation surgery. Patients who describe a phantom sensation or phantom pain should start this type of desensitization as early as possible to help control these feelings. Tapping, rubbing, and massage can initially be done over the Ace wrap and ultimately directly over the skin as the wound heals. Other pain control measures used in physical therapy include rubbing different textures on the skin and electrical stimulation with a transcutaneous electrical nerve stimulation (TENS) unit. A pre-prosthetic therapy program should include mobility activities, such as transfers to a wheelchair; transfers to critical areas, such as toilet areas; car transfers; and high/low transfers to the bed. Most patients should be able to achieve standing and hopping within 3 to 7 days after amputation surgery. Ideally, this can be started with the parallel bars in a therapy department and progress to a walker and crutches as patients improve. Careful cardiopulmonary monitoring is necessary in most patients with diabetes and dysvascular disease. Monitoring of blood sugar levels may be necessary as they often change in the time period immediately after surgery. Proper inspection of the remaining foot is necessary and should be instituted by a treating therapist; education of patients regarding inspection is helpful.

WOUND CARE

All patients with amputations must be assessed for wound care issues. The amputation surgical site itself is essentially a healing wound with sutures or staples in place. In the acute care setting immediately after surgery, a surgeon applies a soft compressive dressing. Once this is removed, daily dressing changes can be instituted. If wound healing seems to be progressing appropriately, the surgical site can be simply covered with a nonstick dressing and appropriate roll gauze applied to cover the surgical site. This is covered with Ace wrapping using a figure-of-eight pattern. If the new amputation site has an open wound that seems unusually delayed, it needs additional attention. The size of the wound should be assessed, including length, width, and depth, the quality of the tissue, and potential infection problems. Infection can be indicated by fever, odor, surrounding erythema, or increasing drainage from this wound. If there is necrotic and nonviable tissue present, it should be removed with sharp débridement using scissors, forceps, and scalpel. Any tissue that is brown, black, or yellow is compromised or nonviable and typically removed with sharp débridement. This can be performed by a treating surgeon or a wound care specialist.

Any open wounds at the amputation site or other locations on the lower limb generally are managed using saline-based dressing. Saline dressings can be in a liquid fashion, hydrogel in a tube or spray, or hydrogel impregnated into gauze. Saline dressings with a silver additive are used to help control infection in addition to systemic antibiotic use.

If a wound cannot be sufficiently débrided, a topical enzyme agent may be helpful for the first 7 to 14 days. Surgical débridement or sharp débridement is preferable but not always possible. A heavily draining wound should be covered with an absorptive dressing, which may include collagen fiber, synthetic fiber, or calcium alginate gauze. These dressings should be changed when they are 50% to 75% saturated. Deeper wounds of a residual limb or remaining leg can be treated with a vacuum-assisted closure device. These devices are applied directly to a wound with negative applied pressure of 60 to 120 mm Hg for approximately 20 hours per day. The vacuum-assisted closure dressings generally are changed 3 times per week. Maintaining appropriate vacuum around the perimeter of the wound is critical. Often, a specialized wound care nurse or wound care physician is necessary to help manage this program. Shallow healing wounds that are less than 2 cm in size should not delay prosthetic fitting or prosthetic therapy program.

Wounds that show signs of infection should be aggressively treated with systemic antibiotics based on deep tissue culture after débridement. Empiric treatment with broad-spectrum antibiotics may be necessary in some circumstances, but a change to a more targeted antibiotic is more appropriate. Patients with diabetes and dysvascular disease are often infected with polymicrobial and mixed aerobic-anaerobic infections, which should be assessed carefully as part of the wound culture process. Once a wound is cleared of infection, wound dressings with a saline-based product can be instituted. A wound that seems to be healing slowly can be treated with a growth factor gel, which may help speed the healing process. If wound healing is delayed due to hypoxia or ischemia in the surrounding area, then further testing, such as transcutaneous oxygen measurement, may be needed. Vascular evaluation of arterial and venous blood flow often is important in patients with delayed wound healing. Every attempt to restore proper arterial inflow and venous outflow should be made to heal a wound and preserve the longest possible amputation limb length. If a wound is hypoxic based on results of transcutaneous oxygen measurement studies, hyperbaric oxygen treatment may be appropriate to improve the healing process and salvage the limb.

PAIN MANAGEMENT

Pain management in the post-operative phase is helpful to allow patients to mobilize rapidly and successfully. Surgical pain is treated with opioids or nonopioids that are tapered rapidly over 7 to 14 days. Other pain management treatment should be instituted, including application of topical anesthetic gels if a surgical site is healed, application of a TENS unit to control nerve pain, and continued use of nonopioids for residual limb pain. All patients should be reassured that phantom sensation is normal after amputation and that no specific treatment is needed.

If patients describe painful or disturbing feelings in the phantom segment (phantom pain), then a variety of treatments are appropriate. Compression with Ace wrap or shrinker often helps with phantom pain and allows patients to regain some control of the pain. Use of TENS may help with phantom pain. Tapping, rubbing, and massaging for desensitization may help with phantom pain. Imagery or use of a mirror to help patients imagine that they are mobilizing these absent segments of the lower limb may help them regain control over these disturbing sensations in the foot and ankle. Medications to control phantom pain also are available (discussed later).

FOOTWEAR

Prevention of injury to the remaining foot is a critical goal for an entire prosthetic team. Assessment of the remaining foot for physical and physiological deficiencies is important. It is common for diabetic/dysvascular patients to have deformities, such as hallux valgus, hammertoes, and prominent metatarsal heads. The presence of peripheral neuropathy indicates that a patient has impairment of sensation and may have atrophy of the intrinsic muscles of the foot due to the underlying neuropathy, making all bony prominences more vulnerable to pressure. The presence of callus on the plantar surface of the foot is an indication of excessive pressure and needs attention and redistribution of pressure. Patients with diabetes and peripheral neuropathy tend to develop a more pes cavus foot deformity due to the intrinsic muscle atrophy, thereby putting pressure at the heel and the metatarsal heads. Only 30% of the available plantar surface takes 100% of the load. Therefore, redistribution of the load to the remainder of the foot using a custom-molded foot orthotic is helpful. Some patients develop plantarflexion contracture, further loading the forefoot and putting the foot at risk for callus and skin breakdown. Extradepth orthopedic shoes have additional room in the rearfoot and forefoot for a custom-molded foot orthotic and for a foot deformity. Orthopedic shoes typically have a strong heel counter, a fairly rigid inner sole, a generous toe box, and a seamless interior. If hammertoes are present, a high toe box may be necessary. If hallux valgus deformity is severe, a bunion last shoe may be appropriate. If there is callusing at the metatarsal heads, use of a metatarsal pad or metatarsal bar may be appropriate to unload the metatarsal heads.

It is preferable to use a custom-molded foot orthotic with a multidensity construction to treat some of the common deformities that occur in patients with diabetes and peripheral neuropathy. Typically, the firmest layer of material goes on the bottom and the softest on top, allowing for supporting and cushioning of the foot. Materials, such as neoprene rubber, therma-cork, and latex, are used as a more rigid base material and are covered with a soft foam top layer. These are fabricated from a cast or foam impression of the foot to help distribute pressure away from high-risk areas and apply it to areas that are more pressure tolerant.

Even with properly fitted extradepth orthopedic shoes and custom-molded foot orthotics, patients are instructed to check their foot and their shoes on a daily basis for any problems or complications. Shoes and molded foot orthotics generally are replaced annually but may require modification or adjustment more frequently.

TIME FRAME OF REHABILITATION

In an ideal setting, patients spend only the first 2 to 5 days in an acute care hospital during the post-operative time period. During this time, residual limb shaping with Ace wrap should be taking place. A pre-prosthetic therapy program of ROM strengthening and mobility should be started 1–2 days after surgery. Patients should be mobilizing out of bed as soon as tolerated. Treatment of pain should take place in this early time period. The next phase, from approximately day 5 through day 21 after surgery, is continued treatment with a pre-prosthetic therapy program. This can take place in a home setting if appropriate services are available or in a subacute rehabilitation setting. If patients have ongoing significant medical problems in addition to amputation, transfer to an acute rehabilitation setting may be medically warranted. This time period is important to continue to aggressively manage pain and improve mobility, strength, and range of motion. This is a high-risk time for patients for developing hip and knee flexor contracture or plantarflexion contractures at the ankle. Patient education should continue throughout this time period, including weekly re-evaluation by a prosthetic team. Regular assessment of the healing and shaping of a residual limb helps to plan for the next phase of prosthetic fitting.

During the third or fourth week after amputation, sutures and staples are removed by a surgical team. At this point, if healing is sufficient, change from an Ace wrap to a shrinker sock is appropriate to help with continued shrinking and shaping. The shrinker is initially applied over a nylon sheath to prevent traction of the surgical site. As the surgical site continues to heal, the shrinker eventually can be pulled directly over the skin. The shrinker should be worn 23 hours per day, but the skin should be checked at least 3 times per day for red areas or irritation. Measurement of the limb at this time is important to monitor shaping of the limb. A transtibial amputation limb should be achieving cylindric shape at this time in preparation for casting of a preliminary prosthesis. Transfemoral amputations may be cone shaped at this point in preparation for prosthetic fitting. Casting for a preliminary prosthesis typically is done between weeks 3 and 5 based on healing and shaping. If there is a wound present, but the wound is smaller than 2 cm and in the healing phase, then it is appropriate to proceed with casting and fitting of a prosthesis. Training with a preliminary prosthesis should start as soon as the device is properly fitted and checked out. A prosthetist and physician should agree that the fitting is appropriate and sufficient to proceed with the therapy program.

The length of a physical therapy program for transtibial amputation during prosthetic training is typically 3 times a week for 4 to 6 weeks to achieve basic mobility goals. Transfemoral amputation may require 6 to 12 weeks of therapy program with the prosthesis to accomplish safe and independent ambulation indoors and outdoors. Use of a preliminary prosthesis continues until patients have accomplished independent ambulation and a residual limb no longer is decreasing in volume. This should be monitored on a monthly basis by a prosthetic team. Patients can be fitted into a permanent prosthesis between 3 and 6 months after amputation once limb shape is stabilized and ambulation has plateaued.[8–13]

ENERGY REQUIREMENTS

There is an increase in energy requirement for ambulation with lower-limb amputation with or without prosthesis. Review of the literature on this subject over the past 30 years shows that there has been variability in results and findings related to the increase in energy requirements at various levels of amputation.[14–18] If patients are required to walk at a fixed speed and compared with normal controls, there is always an increase in energy closely associated with the level of amputation. Patients with long transtibial amputation may have only 10% to 20% increase in energy cost compared with normal controls; however, short transtibial amputation may be up to 30% to 40% increased energy compared with controls. Long transfemoral amputation may require as little as 40% additional energy; however, shorter transfemoral amputation may require as much as 80% additional energy. Hip disarticulation and hemipelvectomy typically have at least 80% additional energy and can be much higher. Bilateral transtibial amputation requires 60 to 80% additional energy over controls. Bilateral transfemoral amputation may require greater than 200% additional energy over normal ambulation. Once patients are sufficiently trained with their permanent prosthesis, their energy requirements may decrease. If patients are allowed to walk at self-selected speed once they are trained with their prosthesis, their energy demand decreases. Patients' self-selected speed with a prosthesis inevitably is much slower than normal ambulation speed.

MEDICARE FUNCTIONAL LEVEL AND PROSTHETIC COMPONENTRY

Evaluation of patients by a physician and prosthetist helps determine a patient's Medicare functional level. These levels were established in 1995 by Medicare as an attempt to guide physicians and prosthetists in providing appropriate componentry for patients' level of function. Based on patients' medical conditions and level of amputation, it is a physician's role to estimate what a patient's functional level will be after fitting of a prosthesis and completion of an appropriate rehabilitation program.

If patients do better or worse than expected, then the Medicare functional level should be changed or adjusted for future prosthetic componentry. A summary of the Medicare functional levels is as follows:

Level 0—bed-bound, non-ambulatory patient
Level I—transfers or household ambulation only
Level II—limited community ambulator who is impaired by distance or obstacles in the community
Level III—unlimited community ambulator who can walk at variable cadence for greater than 400 yards
Level IV—high-energy activities, including work and sports activities

Based on evaluation by a physician and prosthetist, functional level is established and selection of prosthetic feet and knees is dictated by that functional level. For patients who have level 0 or no potential for ambulation, no prosthesis is provided or covered according to Medicare guidelines. For patients at level I, the appropriate foot includes solid ankle, cushion heel (SACH) or single axis because they are level surface ambulators at best. If patients have transfemoral amputation at level I, they can be provided with a locking or stance-controlled knee, which swings at a fixed cadence. Level II ambulators can be provided a multiple-axis foot because they tolerate some outdoor ambulation on uneven terrain. For patients with transfemoral amputation, it is expected that they will continue to ambulate at a fixed cadence. Level II transfemoral patients could be provided a locking knee, stance-controlled knee, or polycentric knee. For patients deemed level III or level IV, a prosthetic foot can include energy storing or dynamic response features to allow patient ambulation for longer distances and at variable speeds. At level III or level IV, for patients with transfemoral amputation, the knee componentry can include hydraulic mechanisms or microprocessor controlled knees to allow variable speed. These Medicare guidelines do not apply to patients with bilateral lower limb amputation, and it is left to the judgment and decision of a physician and prosthetist to provide the appropriate foot and knee componentry for these patients. There are no guidelines from Medicare or any other provider related to the socket design or suspension.

PROSTHETIC DESIGN AND COMPONENTRY

For patients with transtibial amputation, contemporary socket designs include total contact, patellar tendon bearing of the residual limb via a soft interface and rigid frame. The patellar tendon and medial tibial flare area still are used most often to take additional pressure. Less pressure is tolerated at the tibial crest, at the distal and proximal fibula, and the distal tibia. These areas are relieved within the socket to allow less pressure but still maintain gentle contact. All transtibial sockets have some type of soft interface material.

In a preliminary prosthesis, a closed cell foam material (liner) is used to act as a soft interface. This material is desirable because it is easy to modify, such as with grinding or by adding additional pads. As a patient's limb slowly shrinks and matures, frequent modifications are necessary at this stage. There is always a rigid socket over the soft interface, which is usually a thermoplastic or laminated material. Patients generally wear special prosthetic socks over the skin before they apply a prosthesis. As the residual limb shrinks over time, patients continue to add more and more of these socks to accommodate for the volume loss. If excessive perspiration or skin irritation occurs, a specialized sock, called a liner liner sock, can be used, which contains a silver thread that helps control the irritation of the skin and perspiration of the skin within a prosthesis. Patients should be followed up every 2 to 4 weeks by a prosthetist and physician to monitor the fit of the prosthesis and shrinking of the residual limb.

Suspension on a preliminary prosthesis commonly is a supracondylar wedge or elastic sleeve suspension, providing high medial-lateral walls for good medial and lateral stability, yet allowing flexion of the knee from full extension to 90° flexion. Other alternatives for suspension include a supracondylar strap or knee joints with a thigh corset. The connector from the socket to the foot is called a shank or pylon and is typically of a lightweight material, such as titanium or aluminum. The choice of material is based on patient weight and activity level and should be discussed in detail with a prosthetist. The selection of a prosthetic foot is based on a patient activity level (discussed previously). Many patients who were active before amputation resume level III functional activities. There is a multitude of prosthetic feet from a variety of manufacturers and vendors available in this category, including multiaxial feet and energy-storing feet. The decision of prosthetic foot should be made based on patient activity, patient body weight, and discussion between physician and prosthetist.

Once patients have completed fitting and training with a preliminary prosthesis, they proceed to permanent prosthesis. One of the changes that may occur with a permanent prosthesis includes change in the socket design. A permanent transtibial socket still has total contact design with additional pressure at the patellar tendon and at the medial tibial flare. The soft interface, however, may be a gel liner with or without a pin suspension. This design is useful because a patient's residual limb shape should remain consistent for months or years, providing protection for patients with dysvascular skin or irregular shape. The gel liner is applied directly over the skin and creates a negative pressure or suction; the pin at the bottom of the liner mechanically locks to the prosthetic socket. Other options include a gel liner without a pin that is suspended using an auxiliary suspension sleeve outside the socket. There are now suction gel liners that have a flap seal in the lower half that create a vacuum seal from the liner to the socket.

There are active and passive vacuum systems that draw air out of the space between the gel liner and the socket to maintain intimate fit and contact. These active and passive vacuum systems require an airtight seal proximally with a silicon-type elastic sleeve.

The transfemoral amputation socket design on a preliminary prosthesis also incorporates soft prosthetic socks and a socket with a soft interface material and rigid outer frame. The soft inner socket typically is a flexible thermaplastic material that is molded over a cast of a patient's limb, and an outer rigid frame of carbon fiber lamination is fitted over the liner. Patients continue to add prosthetic socks as the residual limb shrinks, and modifications are needed on a regular basis to the inner flexible liner of the prosthesis. The weight-bearing characteristics of the transfemoral socket include total contact of the residual limb with increased pressure at the ischium and gluteal muscle. Containment of the ischium within the posterior/medial socket is critical to minimize any lateral shifting of the socket in stance phase. This is accomplished through a sloped posterior/medial wall that allows the ischium to slide into the socket and remain captured within the socket. The medial/lateral dimension of a contemporary socket is narrower than the anterior and posterior dimension. Suspension of a prosthesis in the preliminary design is usually through an elastic or nonelastic waist belt.

A permanent transfemoral socket incorporates a soft interface and a rigid outer frame. A suction system, however, where a patient's limb slides directly into the soft interface socket, allowing air to expel through a one-way valve in the distal portion of the socket, can be used. No additional waist belt or suspension may be necessary in this case. This may be a wet fit using a lotion on the skin or a dry fit using a special plastic bag to pull the residual limb into the socket. There also are suction gel liners with pin or strap suspension similar to what was available in the transtibial socket design. These provide additional cushioning and protection of a residual limb if necessary.

Active vacuum systems electronically or mechanically expel air from the space between a residual limb and socket to promote containment of the residual limb within the socket. These generally are reserved for patients who are most active.

The selection of a prosthetic knee unit should be based on patient activity level and weight and ultimately on a patient's Medicare functional level. The more sophisticated knees are the heaviest and most complex knees. The microprocessor-controlled knees add a level of safety and security, with an incorporated "stumble recovery" mechanism and recalibration of the knee 50 times per second.

Microprocessor-controlled knees help minimize gait deviations, because they are designed to meet individual gait requirements of patients through computer software that is programmed by a prosthetist. The choice of knee units, is based on the overall patient activity and their medicare functional level. The benefits of a microprocessor-controlled knee sometimes are outweighed by weight or the cost of these devices. Patients who are at highest risk for falls and injury, however, after amputation may be those who benefit the most from a microprocessor-controlled knee. The overall weight of a prosthesis depends on the socket, the interface, the knee, and the foot unit. Patient cardiopulmonary status may dictate how much weight patients can tolerate.[19–22]

PROSTHETIC TRAINING

Once patients are fitted with a preliminary prosthesis, education of patients continues. Prosthetic education starts with a prosthetist and includes a therapist and physician. Proper donning and doffing technique of a prosthesis is learned first. Initial wearing schedule for a prosthesis should be 1 to 2 hours per day with advancement of 1 additional hour each day if tolerated. This should be monitored by a physical therapist, prosthetist or physician. Patients initially start partial weight bearing on a preliminary prosthesis and slowly progress to full weight bearing as tolerated. Training of patients in ambulation with a prosthesis should start at the parallel bars to allow for reciprocal gait. If patients must progress to a walker, certain gait deviations are introduced. Patients who ultimately use a walker long term may be trained with a walker during therapy program; however, patients who progress away from assisted devices should go from the parallel bars directly to forearm crutches, if possible. As they improve, progression to a cane and potentially no assistive device is the ultimate goal. The training time necessary to accomplish this typically is 4 to 6 weeks in transtibial amputees, 6 to 12 weeks in transfemoral amputees, and 12 weeks or more in bilateral lower limb amputees.[23,24] Outpatient physical therapy programs typically take place 3 times per week and there are home exercises and activities that should be incorporated into a daily schedule. Strengthening of the critical muscles in the upper and lower limbs and overall cardiopulmonary conditioning should be part of a therapy program after fitting of a prosthesis. There should be monthly follow-ups by a physician and prosthetist to monitor skin integrity, prosthetic fit, and ambulation status.

Functional goals of prosthetic training should include ambulation on level and unlevel surfaces and progressing to stairs and other more challenging areas. Patients should be able to maneuver from the kitchen, bedroom, and bathroom to accomplish toileting, bathing, and dressing activities independently with a prosthesis. If patients were driving before amputation, the therapy program should address return to driving. If there is amputation of the right lower limb, modification of the vehicle, including a left foot accelerator pedal, may be necessary.

COMPLICATIONS

Unfortunately, morbidity and mortality after lower limb amputation in the older dysvascular population have not changed in decades. The 50/50 rule still applies to morbidity and mortality. There is an approximately 50% survival rate over 5 years after amputation in the older dysvascular population. Of the survivors, up to 50% have a second major amputation during that 5-year time period.[25] In addition, there are intermittent issues with skin irritation or breakdown as volume loss and muscle atrophy occur in a residual limb in the first 5 years. Patients must continue to follow up with a prosthetic team to make modifications and adjustments to accommodate volume changes. Patients must be monitored for ongoing cardiopulmonary status as they age. Periodic assessment for hip and knee range of motion and strength is important to make sure patients are maintaining sufficient strength and range of motion to control the prosthetic device as originally designed. If congestive heart failure or renal failure arises, then volume of a residual limb may change frequently. If limb volume cannot be controlled medically or mechanically, the prosthesis must be accommodated for the larger size of the residual limb. If patients have some days when a residual limb is larger and other days when the limb is smaller, the prosthesis must be fitted for the larger size. Additional socks can be applied on days when a residual limb is smaller. Patients are encouraged to continue use of a shrinker sock at night, when the prosthesis is removed, to try to control residual limb volume consistently day after day.

Patients often change weight as they age or as their social situations change. If there is a sudden change, such as loss of a family member or spouse, which may leave patients alone in their home, then nutrition and dietary habits often may change. The availability of food shopping and meal preparation may have changed dramatically. Depression may set in and cause a change in patients' interest in food. Therefore, regular monitoring of patients' weight is critical during these times. Patients should have their weight checked on a regular basis when they come for prosthetic follow-up and more frequently when they go though traumatic social changes. Patients should be followed every 6 to 12 months while they are in their permanent prosthesis or more frequently if they are having medical issues.

Falls are common in the elderly and more common in the disabled elderly dysvascular population. An amputation increases the risk of falls. Most falls are preventable if appropriate assistive devices and instructions are provided. Balance and vision may be compromised as patients age, and, hopefully, these can be compensated through provision of assistive devices and possible retraining in physical therapy.

Additional care in the home may be necessary for nighttime activities when lighting is poor and depth perception may be further impaired. The ultimate goal is to allow continued safe ambulation of amputee patients indoors and outdoors as tolerated, with or without their prosthetic device.

SUMMARY

The rehabilitation management of diabetic patients with amputation is complicated by the comorbidities associated with diabetes. Delays in wound healing, cardiopulmonary compromise, and peripheral neuropathy are some of the many issues taken into account when assessing this patient population. The impact of these medical issues on patients' functional status before amputation provides some of the most valuable information in formulating the rehabilitation program after amputation. Thorough history and physical examination are still the cornerstone for planning a safe and effective treatment program. Setting realistic goals for a treatment program helps an entire team work toward an endpoint and avoids any unrealistic expectations. Precautions must be taken to carefully monitor patient performance and tolerance during the rehabilitation phase of their care. Proper selection of prosthetic design and components help maximize the functional outcome rather than hinder it. Regular follow-up and long-term management of diabetic patients with amputation help to maintain the functional goals achieved as long as possible.

REFERENCES

1. van Velzen JM, van Bennekom CA, Polomski W, et al. Physical capacity and walking ability after lower limb amputation: a systematic review. Clin Rehabil 2006;20(11):999–1016 Review. PubMed PMID: 17065543.
2. Gailey R, Allen K, Castles J, et al. Review of secondary physical conditions associated with lower-limb amputation and long-term prosthesis use. J Rehabil R D 2008;45(1):15–29 Review. PubMed PMID: 18566923.
3. Ingham SJ, Chamlian TR, de Souza JM, et al. Transitory myocardial ischemia in patients with vascular lower limb amputation: relationship with long-term atherothrombotic events. Am J Phys Med Rehabil 2009;88(2):114–8. PubMed PMID: 19169177.
4. Meulenbelt HE, Geertzen JH, Jonkman MF, et al. Determinants of skin problems of the stump in lower-limb amputees. Arch Phys Med Rehabil 2009;90(1):74–81 PubMed PMID: 19154832.
5. Stepien JM, Cavenett S, Taylor L, et al. Activity levels among lower-limb amputees: self-report versus step activity monitor. Arch Phys Med Rehabil 2007; 88(7):896–900. PubMed PMID: 17601471.
6. Goldberg T. Postoperative management of lower extremity amputations. Phys Med Rehabil Clin N Am 2006;17(1):173–80, vii. Review. PubMed PMID: 16517350.
7. van Velzen AD, Nederhand MJ, Emmelot CH, et al. Early treatment of trans-tibial amputees: retrospective analysis of early fitting and elastic bandaging. Prosthet Orthot Int 2005;29(1):3–12. PubMed PMID: 16180373.
8. Zidarov D, Swaine B, Gauthier-Gagnon C. Quality of life of persons with lower-limb amputation during rehabilitation and at 3-month follow-up. Arch Phys Med Rehabil 2009;90(4):634–45. PubMed PMID: 19345780.
9. Vanross ER, Johnson S, Abbott CA. Effects of early mobilization on unhealed dysvascular transtibial amputation stumps: a clinical trial. Arch Phys Med Rehabil 2009;90(4):610–7. PubMed PMID: 19345776.
10. Stineman MG, Kwong PL, Kurichi JE, et al. The effectiveness of inpatient rehabilitation in the acute postoperative phase of care after transtibial or transfemoral amputation: study of an integrated health care delivery system. Arch Phys Med Rehabil 2008;89(10):1863–72. PubMed PMID: 18929014.
11. Cumming JC, Barr S, Howe TE. Prosthetic rehabilitation for older dysvascular people following a unilateral transfemoral amputation. Cochrane Database Syst Rev 2006;(4):CD005260. Review. PubMed PMID: 17054250.
12. Trower TA. Changes in lower extremity prosthetic practice. Phys Med Rehabil Clin N Am 2006;17(1):23–30, v-vi. Review. PubMed PMID: 16517343.

13. Dillingham TR, Pezzin LE. Rehabilitation setting and associated mortality and medical stability among persons with amputations. Arch Phys Med Rehabil 2008;89(6):1038–45. PubMed PMID: 18503797.
14. Wu YJ, Chen SY, Lin MC, et al. Energy expenditure of wheeling and walking during prosthetic rehabilitation in a woman with bilateral transfemoral amputations. Arch Phys Med Rehabil 2001;82(2):265–9. PubMed PMID: 11239324.
15. Cutson TM, Bongiorni DR. Rehabilitation of the older lower limb amputee: a brief review. J Am Geriatr Soc 1996;44(11):1388–93 Review. PubMed PMID: 8909359.
16. Hagberg K, Haggstrom E, Branemark R. Physiological cost index (PCI) and walking performance in individuals with transfemoral prostheses compared to healthy controls. Disabil Rehabil 2007;29(8):643–9. PubMed PMID:17453985.
17. Graham LE, Datta D, Heller B, et al. A comparative study of oxygen consumption for conventional and energy-storing prosthetic feet in transfemoral amputees. Clin Rehabil 2008;22(10–11):896–901. PubMed PMID: 18955421.
18. Vanicek N, Strike S, McNaughton L, et al. Gait patterns in transtibial amputee fallers vs. non-fallers: biomechanical differences during level walking. Gait Posture 2009;29(3):415–20. Epub 2008 Dec 13. PubMed PMID: 19071021.
19. Zmitrewicz RJ, Neptune RR, Walden JG, et al. The effect of foot and ankle prosthetic components on braking and propulsive impulses during transtibial amputee gait. Arch Phys Med Rehabil 2006;87(10):1334–9. PubMed PMID: 17023242.
20. Klute GK, Berge JS, Orendurff MS, et al. Prosthetic intervention effects on activity of lower-extremity amputees. Arch Phys Med Rehabil 2006;87(5):717–22. PubMed PMID: 16635636.
21. Nelson VS, Flood KM, Bryant PR, et al. Limb deficiency and prosthetic management. 1. Decision making in prosthetic prescription and management. Arch Phys Med Rehabil 2006;87(3 Suppl 1):S3–9 Review. PubMed PMID: 16500187.
22. Kaufman KR, Levine JA, Brey RH, et al. Energy expenditure and activity of transfemoral amputees using mechanical and microprocessor-controlled prosthetic knees. Arch Phys Med Rehabil 2008;89(7):1380–5. PubMed PMID: 18586142; PubMed Central PMCID: PMC2692755.
23. Su PF, Gard SA, Lipschutz RD, et al. Differences in gait characteristics between persons with bilateral transtibial amputations, due to peripheral vascular disease and trauma, and able-bodied ambulators. Arch Phys Med Rehabil 2008;89(7): 1386–94. PubMed PMID: 18586143.
24. Su PF, Gard SA, Lipschutz RD, et al. Gait characteristics of persons with bilateral transtibial amputations. J Rehabil R D 2007;44(4):491–501. PubMed PMID: 18247246.
25. Kulkarni J, Pande S, Morris J. Survival rates in dysvascular lower limb amputees. Int J Surg 2006;4(4):217–21. Epub 2006 Aug 14. PubMed PMID: 17462354.

Psychosocial Factors in Chronic Pain in the Dysvascular and Diabetic Patient

Katherine A. Raichle, PhD[a,b,*], Travis L. Osborne, PhD[a,c],
Mark P. Jensen, PhD[a,d]

KEYWORDS

- Dysvascular • Pain • Chronic
- Biophysical • Coping • Psychologies

PAIN IN DYSVASCULAR AND DIABETIC PATIENTS

Dysvascular and diabetic patients are faced with high rates of chronic pain as a conse-quence of numerous secondary sequelae, such as diabetic neuropathy and limb loss, to name 2 of the most common. Diabetic peripheral neuropathy (DPN) accounts for the most common of all of the diabetic neuropathies, explaining approximately 78% of those with any type of diabetic neuropathy.[1,2] The rates of those with painful DPN are as high as 12% to 15%,[1] with this pain usually described as having burning, elec-tric, sharp, shooting, tingling, and lancinating qualities.[3] There is no cure for DPN, but treatment may include maintaining glycemic control and use of certain antidepres-sants, antiepileptics, and opioids.[4] Unfortunately, medication often must be dosed at lower than optimum levels to minimize the unpleasant side effects of these drugs, limiting the effectiveness of these medications to treat pain.[5]

In a recent study, Ziegler-Graham and colleagues[6] found that in 2005, about 38% of all 1.6 million persons living with a limb loss had an amputation secondary to

---

This work was supported by grant #H133B980017 from the Department of Education's National Institute of Disability and Rehabilitation Research and grant "Management of Chronic Pain in Rehabilitation" PO1 HD33988, from the National Institute of Child Health and Human Develop-ment, National Center for Medical Rehabilitation Research, National Institutes of Health.

[a] Department of Rehabilitation Medicine, University of Washington School of Medicine, Box 356490, 1959 Pacific St. NE, Seattle, WA 98195-6490, USA
[b] Department of Psychology, Seattle University, 901 12th Avenue, Pavilion 120, Seattle, WA 98122, USA
[c] Anxiety & Stress Reduction Center of Seattle (ASRC), 1218 Third Avenue, Suite #500, Seattle, WA 9810, USA
[d] Multidisciplinary Pain Center, University of Washington Medical Center—Roosevelt, 4245 Roosevelt Way Northeast, Seattle, WA 98105-6920, USA
* Corresponding author.
E-mail address: raichlek@u.washington.edu (K. A. Raichle).

Phys Med Rehabil Clin N Am 20 (2009) 705–717
doi:10.1016/j.pmr.2009.06.005
1047-9651/09/$ – see front matter © 2009 Elsevier Inc. All rights reserved.

dysvascular disease with a comorbid diagnosis of diabetes mellitus. Numerous studies have shown that chronic pain in multiple sites is common for persons with an acquired amputation, with phantom limb pain (PLP), residual limb pain (RLP), and back pain reflecting 3 of the most common areas of difficulty.[7,8] In another recent survey, Ephraim and colleagues[7] found that, of 914 persons with amputation sampled, 80% reported PLP, 68% reported RLP, and 62% reported back pain, compared with the 12% to 45% rate of back pain for the general population. Moreover, 39% and 30% of their sample rated PLP and RLP as severe (ie, having an average intensity of 7 or more on a 0–10 scale), respectively. Unfortunately, similar to DPN, PLP and RLP are often refractory to treatment.[9]

Taken together, the prevalence of common types of chronic pain in dysvascular and diabetic patients coupled with the refractory nature of this pain calls for an approach to chronic pain management that also considers psychological and social factors that impact pain and related dysfunction; that is, a biopsychosocial approach.

PSYCHOSOCIAL FACTORS IN CHRONIC PAIN

Researchers and scientists have put forth a tremendous amount of effort to understand the complex nature of pain. The emergent understanding of anatomy and sensory physiology within the past century has fueled an initial focus of understanding pain from a neurologic and biochemical perspective. This approach, the biomedical model, has centered our attention on the processing of peripheral noxious sensory input in the central nervous system. Under the tenets of this model, reports of pain sensations lead to a search for pathology or physical injury and to the development of treatments geared toward symptom reduction. Although the biologic underpinnings of pain are an important piece of the puzzle, restrictive biomedical models have been unable to adequately explain all aspects of pain, including differential outcomes to similar pain treatments, the variable association between impairment, reported pain intensity and disability, and the development and maintenance of chronic pain in the absence of identifiable pathology. In consequence, our attempt to understand pain has broadened beyond the scope of a purely biologic model.[10] Over the past few decades, the field has moved toward an understanding of pain as a process involving the dynamic interaction of biologic, psychological, behavioral, and social variables. This article provides a brief overview of several psychosocial processes, cognitive, affective, and behavioral, that have emerged as influential to the experience, impact, and treatment of pain.

APPRAISALS AND COPING

Of particular interest in the conceptualization of pain as a multidimensional process are the effects of cognitive and behavioral processes on pain and adjustment to pain. An increasing body of research has established the important role that these entities play in the expression of pain and disability.[11,12] This section systematically discusses appraisals and coping repertoires that have emerged as particularly important with regard to their influence on pain behavior, functional limitations, mental health, and adjustment to and perception of pain.

Fear of Movement/Reinjury

Several models have been developed in an attempt to explain why some individuals develop a chronic pain syndrome long after tissue damage or pathology has healed. Lethem and colleagues[13] proposed the Fear-Avoidance Model of Exaggerated Pain to understand why some persons with musculoskeletal pain have an "exaggerated" pain perception that they hypothesized ultimately contributes to functional limitations, development and maintenance of chronic pain, and poorer psychological health. More recently, Vlaeyen and colleagues[14,15] proposed a "cognitive model of fear of move-ment/(re)injury" that is an adaptation of Lethem and colleagues' model. The central tenet of both theories is "fear of pain." Two very different possible responses to this fear are "confrontation" and "avoidance," which are thought to result in a reduction of fear or a maintenance and exacerbation of fear over time, respectively. "Confronta-tion" was hypothesized to contribute to the reintroduction of social and physical activities as the organic etiology of the pain resolves, whereas "avoidance" serves to limit mobility through an avoidance of activities and an exaggerated perception of pain.

Pain-related fear has been examined mostly in persons with acute low back pain, and has been associated with impaired physical performance[14,16] and increased self-reported disability[15-17] beyond that predicted by pain severity and biomedical findings. Pain-related fear has also been examined more recently in persons with sickle-cell disease, with reported rates comparable to those with acute low back pain[18] and persons with pathologic shoulder pain.[19] Pain-related fear has been linked with disability, depressed mood, pain severity, and lower treadmill performance in persons with fibromyalgia syndrome.[20] Finally, the impact of pain-related fear has been found also to contribute significantly to outcomes from delayed-onset shoulder soreness in healthy persons.[21]

Vlaeyen and Linton[22] proposed several pathways by which pain-related fear can lead to disability, decreased activity, and consequent chronic pain in persons with musculoskeletal pain. They synthesized several models, including the aforementioned cognitive model of fear of movement/(re)injury,[14,15] as well as those of Lethem and colleagues,[13] Philips (1987),[23] and Wadell and colleagues.[24] First, it is possible that negative appraisals or beliefs about pain (eg, pain is an indication of injury; expectan-cies of suffering) precipitate the development of pain-related fear. These indices have the potential to contribute disproportionately to disability and adjustment. For example, the belief that one's pain is an ongoing indication of tissue damage or illness, versus that of a stable problem that may improve, can contribute to the avoidance of painful activities. In turn, according to operant models of conditioning (see section on Operant model of pain and illness behaviors), avoidance behaviors are reinforced by repeatedly averting potential opportunities to experience pain. There is little opportu-nity to challenge the belief that pain is an indication of danger to physical health or of acute damage, thus providing no opportunities to reinforce more adaptive beliefs. Over time, maladaptive beliefs can be reinforced and are hypothesized to lead to increased disability.[25] Second, long-standing avoidance of behavior can have a detri-mental impact on musculoskeletal and cardiovascular integrity, possibly resulting in "disuse syndrome."[26] So the perpetuation of avoidance behavior beyond normal heal-ing time can lead to physical deconditioning, thus introducing further obstacles to regaining functional capabilities.[27] Finally, pain-related fear, similar to other types of anxiety, can interfere with cognitive processes and distract from active and adaptive coping. In other words, persons with greater fear avoidance may show heightened awareness to signals of threat and thus pay greater attention to pain-related informa-tion, to the detriment of active coping (see section on Pain-Related Coping).

Treatment studies further corroborate the relationship between pain-related fear and disability. Recent treatments have been successful at reducing pain-related fear and improving functional abilities.[28-30] For example, Boersma and colleagues[30] evaluated the effectiveness of in vivo exposure to reduce maladaptive beliefs and expectations and increase functioning in persons with back pain. Through graded exposure to ordinary movements and activities, they recorded a decrease in fear and avoidance beliefs and subsequent increase in overall functioning. Moreover, in the context of a multidisciplinary pain treatment program, Jensen and colleagues[31] found that decreases in the belief that pain signals damage was associated with decreases in patient disability. Taken together, these treatment studies substantiate the potential detrimental impact of pain-related fear and lend support for the utility of targeting this factor in treatment.

Pain-Related Coping

Pain-related coping strategies, including cognitive and behavioral efforts to deal with and attempt to reduce or minimize pain, play a central role in predicting disability and adjustment to pain. A myriad of coping strategies have been shown to influence the perception of pain intensity, the ability to manage or endure pain, and one's ability to persist with activities of daily living.[32] Coping strategies that have been examined include praying/hoping, ignoring pain, distraction, resting, task persistence, guarding, asking for assistance, relaxation, positive coping self-statements, exercise/strength, seeking social support, and pacing, to name only a few. It is outside the scope of this article to review the body of research that has examined each of these coping responses,[32] thus the authors focus on a few that seem to be particularly influential in the prediction of adjustment in persons with pain.

Broadly speaking, coping strategies can be divided between those that are active versus those that are passive. Active coping strategies (eg, exercise, distraction, ignoring pain) are more consistently associated with better psychological and functional outcomes, whereas passive coping strategies (eg, withdrawal, resting, guarding, medication use) generally predict inferior outcomes.[33] The passive coping responses that seem to be most detrimental are resting in response to pain and guarding painful body parts, both of which have been linked with poor adjustment and disability in persons with chronic pain,[34–37] as well as PLP.[38] In a recent longitudinal study, Steultjens and colleagues[39] found that resting predicted disability 3 months later for persons with knee osteoarthritis. Alternatively, active coping strategies, including pacing and exercise, seem to be associated with better psychological and functional outcomes.[40,41] Because of the correlational nature of these studies, it is not possible to draw conclusions regarding the extent to which coping plays a causal role in the adjustment to pain. To identify the mechanisms that promote changes in strategies of coping, studies are needed that focus on changing specific coping strategies and observe subsequent changes in outcome.

Of note is the finding that the relationship between detrimental coping strategies (eg, resting) and poor outcomes (eg, functional limitations) is stronger than the relationships between adaptive coping responses and positive outcomes. Maladaptive coping may thus pose a far greater threat to outcome than do adaptive coping strategies in producing positive outcomes. Therefore, interventions that discourage the use of maladaptive coping strategies (eg, discouraging resting and guarding in response to pain, promoting activity) may prove more effective in buffering against disability and functional limitations than interventions that teach and encourage adaptive coping responses.

Catastrophizing

Of particular interest in the domain of appraisals and coping, and the focus of considerable research, is catastrophizing. Catastrophizing can best be characterized as the use of excessive and unrealistic negative self-statements in response to pain, such as, "This pain is awful and I believe that it overwhelms me," or "I can't stand this."[32]

Some investigators have argued that catastrophizing is a type of appraisal, whereas others characterize it as a particular type of (maladaptive) coping. No matter how catastrophizing is conceptualized, however, all agree that it is strongly linked to adjustment for persons with chronic pain. For example, catastrophizing has been consistently associated with increased pain intensity, greater disability and pain-related interference, and poor mental health in a wide variety of pain populations,[31,38,42–45] as well as greater use of analgesics[46] and health care services.[47] Moreover, catastrophizing responses show consistently strong relationships with distress and physical disability of persons with equivalent levels of pain intensity.[48] Turner and colleagues[49] found that among 174 community residents with spinal cord injury and chronic pain, catastrophizing was independently and significantly predictive of psychological distress and pain-related disability above and beyond other coping indices and behavioral responses to pain. Finally, longitudinal research has shown that catastrophizing is able to predict greater pain intensity, functional impairment, and depression 6 months later.[42] In a more recent longitudinal study, catastrophizing has been shown to predict the development of PLP 6 months after amputation in patients with dysvascular disease.[50]

Unfortunately, much of the research on catastrophizing is correlational in nature; the extent to which catastrophizing merely mirrors dysfunction, as opposed to causing dysfunction, is not entirely clear. However, in a recent study catastrophizing was shown to partially mediate the relationship between life stress and depression in a sample of workers' compensation patients with chronic pain, and to be a risk factor for the development of depression following injury.[50]

Another issue concerning catastrophizing is the extent to which it can be differentiated from depression.[51,52] However, the current consensus is that catastrophizing responses are closely linked with, but conceptually distinct from, depression.[47,53] In sum, catastrophizing seems to be one of the strongest predictors of adjustment, experience, and disability related to chronic pain. Whether this strong link is due to a causal impact of catastrophizing on functioning has not yet been determined, and requires causal research.[54]

DEPRESSION AND PAIN

A large body of research has noted and sought to understand the close link between pain, pain interference, and depression.[55–58] One review identified studies with the most stringent criteria for depression, using *Diagnostic and Statistical Manual of Mental Disorders* criteria for Major Depressive Disorder (MDD), and found that between 30% and 54% of persons with chronic pain also meet criteria for MDD.[57] In contrast, the population prevalence rates for current and lifetime major depression are about 5% and 17%, respectively.[59] Fishbain and colleagues[60] sited higher prevalence of suicidal ideation, as well as more suicide attempts in a community sample of patients with pain versus those without. Moreover, depression in persons with chronic pain seems to occur more frequently than in other illness populations, including patients with cardiac disease, cancer, diabetes, and neurologic disorders.[57,61]

The additive impact that concurrent depression has on clinical outcomes of persons with pain has been well documented. Several correlational studies have shown a positive relationship between depression and levels of pain.[62,63] In one review, Bair and colleagues[56] evaluated the outcomes of persons with and without depression treated for pain in managed care and primary care settings. These investigators found across studies that patients with pain and comorbid depression expressed more complaints of pain, greater pain intensity, longer pain duration, and higher rates of persistent pain. In addition, the presence of depression predicted future episodes of pain, including low back, chest, headache, and musculoskeletal pain.[64] Patients with both pain and depression reported greater functional limitations, (eg, mobility, activity restrictions), subsequent days ill in bed, and number of hospitalizations. Finally, Bair and colleagues cited several studies documenting higher unemployment rates and lowered patient satisfaction for those with comorbid pain and depression. Linton,[65] in a review of factors associated with back and neck pain, suggested that psychological factors, including depression, play a more important role in the development of chronic pain problems and disability than biomedical or biochemical factors.

The high rates of depression in persons with chronic pain, as well as the additive detriment of comorbid depression and pain on outcome, has inspired an investigation of the exact nature of this relationship. Although the pain-depression relationship is likely not direct, nor consistently unidirectional, recent progress has been made to understand their temporal relationship, suggesting that depression is a common (but not necessarily universal) consequence of chronic pain.[57,60] Banks and Kerns[57] proposed a diathesis-stress model of a temporal relationship between pain and depression. According to their model the diathesis may be psychological in nature, and include maladaptive schemas or a depressive attributional style that, when combined with the stress associated with the experience of chronic pain, can result in depression. Fishbain and colleagues[60] reviewed 40 studies addressing the relationship between pain and depression, and concluded that a diathesis-stress model is appropriate to explain the relationship. They found support for 3 hypotheses, including (1) depression can be a consequence of pain, (2) certain cognitions (eg, catastrophizing) mediate the relationship between pain and depression, and (3) previous history of depression can predispose an individual with chronic pain to develop depression.

It is outside the scope of this article to explore all of the factors that likely contribute to the development of depression in the context of chronic pain (eg, previous history of depression). Rather, the remainder of this section focuses on a select number of psychosocial mediators that have been most consistently associated with the onset of depression in the context of chronic pain. These mediators include catastrophizing, social support, and pain-related self-efficacy.

As discussed earlier, catastrophizing (eg, an excessive and unrealistically negative appraisals of pain; see previous section) has emerged as a particularly potent cognitive error linked consistently with functional and psychological outcomes in persons with chronic pain[32,47] and is believed specifically to be a possible mediator between pain and depression. In correlational studies, greater catastrophizing has been associated with depression in persons with chronic low back pain[66] and rheumatoid arthritis[42,67] beyond clinical indices. Moreover, in a longitudinal study Keefe and colleagues[42] examined the relationship between catastrophizing and adjustment to chronic pain in persons with rheumatoid arthritis. Greater initial pain-related catastrophizing scores were related with depression, pain intensity, and physical disability 6 months later, after controlling for demographic variables and duration of pain. Smith and colleagues[68] replicated this in a 4-year study of rheumatoid arthritis patients, predicting depression from initial levels of cognitive distortion. Further implicating the mediating role of catastrophic thinking is the success of cognitive behavioral therapy, targeting maladaptive thinking (eg, catastrophizing) in reducing pain and depression in patients with chronic pain.[69]

Pain-related low self-efficacy (eg, lack of confidence in one's own ability to manage, cope with, and function despite persistent pain) has also emerged as a possible mediator between pain, pain interference, and depression. Rudy and colleagues[70] used structural equation modeling with latent variables to examine loss of control and interference in activities as mediators between pain and the development of depression.

Their model provided evidence for the mediation of these factors, and suggested that depression is secondary not to pain but to appraisals about pain. In another cross-sectional study of patients with chronic pain without a prior history of depression, Arnstein and colleagues[71] found support for a mediating role for self-efficacy in predicting depression as well as disability.

The quality and quantity of social support has also been identified as a factor related to depression in persons with chronic pain. In general, a lack of social support has been associated with the occurrence and severity of depression in physical disorders such as chronic pain.[62,72] Romano and colleagues[73] found that persons in families characterized by low cohesion and high conflict reported higher levels of depression. Marital conflict and dissatisfaction have also been linked with depression and adaptation to pain. For example, rheumatoid arthritis patients who report critical responses from spouses also report higher levels of depression.[69] Again, treatment outcome studies lend further evidence to this relationship, as those interventions including spouses and caregivers of persons with pain have been effective in reducing psychological distress and pain.[69]

It is well accepted that depression is disproportionately prevalent in persons with chronic pain compared with other medical populations and in the general public. What is equivocal is the nature and direction of this relationship. The aforementioned mediators, taken together, support the hypothesis that depression is more often a consequence than an antecedent of pain. However, the direction of the pain-depression relationship is unlikely consistently unidirectional, nor is this relationship influenced by psychosocial factors alone (see Bair and colleagues[56] for a review, eg, of common biologic pathways for pain and depression). However, the findings from research highlight the potential importance of psychological factors when considering approaches to the treatment or prevention of depression in the context of pain (see Campbell and colleagues[69] for a review of psychosocial and pharmacologic treatments of depression in persons with pain).

OPERANT MODEL OF PAIN AND ILLNESS BEHAVIORS

The operant model of pain behavior underscores the potential impact of reinforcement contingencies on pain behaviors and the consequent impact on functioning. Operant theory was originally posited by Skinner[74] and is based on the idea that overt behaviors can be altered through environmental contingencies. In theory, behaviors that are reinforced occur more frequently and are maintained over time, whereas those that are punished are decreased in frequency or extinguished. Reinforcement can involve receiving a desired consequence (positive reinforcement) as well as the removal of an undesirable consequence (negative reinforcement), whereas punishment involves receiving an undesired consequence. This theory also posits that when a neutral stimulus is frequently paired with a target behavior and the consequence for this behavior (ie, reinforcement or punishment), it can become a discriminative stimulus that can itself influence the target behavior. Thus, the key to understanding what maintains specific behaviors often involves understanding the discriminative stimuli that actively maintain these behaviors.

Fordyce[27] defined pain behaviors as observable behaviors displayed by persons in pain, including groaning, rubbing, wincing, inactivity, or lying down. He originally applied operant principles to pain behavior suggesting that each can, and often do, come under the control of social reinforcers. According to his application of operant theory, pain behaviors that are initially a response to noxious sensory experience can be reinforced and ultimately maintained by environmental contingencies, long after acute healing and independent of pain. For example, as previously discussed (see section on Fear of Movement/Reinjury), avoidance of undesirable activities or those perceived to induce pain is reinforced independently of pain perception. The nonoccurrence of pain, resulting from avoidance of potentially painful activities, becomes the reinforcement contingency, versus the noxious sensory experience itself.

Operant factors can have an indirect effect on pain as well as on pain behaviors. For example, certain pain behaviors deemed integral to the process of healing can be reinforced by continual avoidance of pain. Limping may be necessary for healing following injury of a lower limb. However, continued reinforcement of this behavior (eg, through avoidance of pain) may result in an altered or distorted ambulatory gate. As a consequence, noxious sensory stimulation may stem from compromised muscles groups.[75] In addition, as discussed earlier in this article, avoidance of activities can result in general physical deconditioning. Deconditioning compromises physical integrity, possibly increasing input of noxious sensory stimulation and perpetuating disability.[75]

There exist several possible sources for reinforcement and perpetuation of pain behaviors, including financial gain, attention and affection from spouse and care givers, attention from health care providers, use of pain medication, and socially sanctioned time out from stressful activities. Fordyce and colleagues[27,76] first emphasized the potential impact that family members can have on reinforcing pain behaviors, suggesting that loved ones are more likely to attend to the patient when pain is reported or displayed, often ignoring the patient during times of wellness. His theory has been corroborated by the work of several researchers who have linked solicitous responding by spouses (eg, responding to overt expressions of pain by offering help or assistance) to poor functional outcomes[77,78] and more severe reports of pain intensity.[79,80]

The tenets of this model have also been supported by the success of treatments for chronic pain that have used the basic principles of operant conditioning. The outcome of such treatments includes reduced interference in social role functioning (ie, work, leisure, marital, family), expression of pain behaviors, pain experience (ie, ratings of intensity, sensation, and unpleasantness), and positive impact on mood/affect (see review by Morley and colleagues[81]). The success of treatment programs based on the tenets of the operant model of pain has implications for clinical practice. For example, clinicians would be advised to avoid focusing on pain severity. Alternatively, asking about and paying attention to activity (ie, exercise, chores, hobbies, work for pay or not, home care), including plans to maintain activity, may influence functional outcomes. In light of the potential impact of family members and care givers, it may prove beneficial to meet with a spouse or significant other and enlist support for reactivation.

Operant factors likely play a central role in precipitating and maintaining disability. Treatment programs based on the tenets of this model have been developed and proven effective for optimizing functional outcomes and psychological health. However, this model has been criticized as oversimplifying the experience of pain. Critics have more recently suggested that operant models of pain behavior constitute only one possible factor contributing to functional outcomes for persons with chronic pain. It is therefore important to be aware that the presence of reinforcement does not mean patients are making up (malingering) or exaggerating symptoms. As stated throughout this article, pain is also likely influenced by cognitive, emotional, social, and biologic factors, as well as the subjective experience of pain.[12]

SUMMARY

In this article several key psychosocial factors that have emerged as predictors of disability and chronic pain are discussed, including cognitive, behavioral, and affective components. Treatment plans should incorporate interventions to address the aforementioned problems, as they provide a proven alternative to pain-focused interventions that have not been effective for the patient.

REFERENCES

1. Dyck PJ, Kratz KM, Karnes JL, et al. The prevalence by staged severity of various types of diabetic neuropathy, retinopathy, and nephropathy in a population-based cohort: the Rochester Diabetic Neuropathy study. Neurology 1993;43(4):817–24.
2. Benbow SJ, MacFarlane IA. Painful diabetic neuropathy. Baillieres Best Pract Res Clin Endocrinol Metab 1999;13(2):295–308.
3. Galer BS, Gianas A, Jensen MP. Painful diabetic polyneuropathy: epidemiology, pain description, and quality of life. Diabetes Res Clin Pract 2000;47(2):123–8.
4. Barbano R, Hart-Gouleau S, Pennella-Vaughan, et al. Pharmacotherapy of painful diabetic neuropathy. Curr Pain Headache Rep 2003;7(3):169–77.
5. Gore M, Bandenburg NA, Dukes E, et al. Pain severity in diabetic peripheral neuropathy is associated with patient functioning, symptom levels of anxiety and depression and sleep. J Pain Symptom Manage 2005;30(4):374–85.
6. Ziegler-Graham K, MacKenzie E, Ephraim P, et al. Estimating the prevalence of limb loss in the United States: 2005 to 2050. Arch Phys Med Rehabil 2008; 89(3):422–9.
7. Ephraim P, Wegener S, MacKenzie E, et al. Phantom pain, residual limb pain, and back pain in amputees: results of a national Survey. Arch Phys Med Rehabil 2005; 86(10):1910–9.
8. Ehde D, Czerniecki J, Smith D, et al. Chronic phantom sensations, phantom pain, residual limb pain, and other regional pain after lower limb amputation. Arch Phys Med Rehabil 2000;81(8):1039–44.
9. Sherman RA. Phantom pain. New York: Plenum Press; 1997.
10. Novy DM, Nelson DV, Francis DJ, et al. Perspectives of chronic pain: an evaluative comparison of restrictive and comprehensive models. Psychol Bull 1995; 118(2):238–47.
11. Chapman CR, Nakamura Y, Flores LY. Chronic pain and consciousness: a constructivist perspective. In: Gatchel RJ, Turk DC, editors. Psychosocial factors in pain: critical perspectives. New York: The Guilford Press; 1999. p. 35–55.
12. Turk DC, Flor H. Chronic pain: a biobehavioral perspective. In: Gatchel RJ, Turk DC, editors. Psychosocial factors in pain: critical perspectives. New York: The Guilford Press; 1999. p. 18–34.
13. Lethem J, Slade PD, Troup JDG, et al. Outline of a fear-avoidance model of exaggerated pain perceptions. Behav Res Ther 1983;21:401–8.
14. Vlaeyen JW, Haazen IW, Schuerman JA, et al. Behavioural rehabilitation of chronic low back pain: comparison of an operant treatment, an operant-cognitive treatment and an operant-respondent treatment. Br J Clin Psychol 1995;34(Pt 1): 95–118.
15. Vlaeyen JW, Kole-Snijders AM, Boeren RG, et al. Fear of movement/(re)injury in chronic low back pain and its relation to behavioral performance. Pain 1995; 62(3):363–72.
16. Crombez G, Eccleston C, Baeyens F, et al. Attention to chronic pain is dependent upon pain-related fear. J Psychosom Res 1999;47(5):403–10.

17. Asmundson GJ, Norton GR, Allerdings MD. Fear and avoidance in dysfunctional chronic back pain patients. Pain 1997;69(3):231–6.

18. Pells J, Edwards C, McDougald CS. Fear of movement (kinesiophobia), pain, and psychopathology in patients with sickle cell disease. Clin J Pain 2007;23(8): 707–13.

19. Huis't Veld RM, Rianne MHA, Vollenbroek-Hutten M, et al. The role of the fear-avoidance model in female workers with neck-shoulder pain related to computer work. Clin J Pain 2007;23:28–34.

20. Turk DC, Robinson JP, Burwinkle T. Prevalence of fear of pain and activity in patients with fibromyalgia syndrome. J Pain 2004;5(9):483–90.

21. George SZ, Dover GC, Fillingim RB. Fear of pain influences outcomes after exercise-induced delayed onset muscle soreness at the shoulder. Clin J Pain 2007; 23(1):76–84.

22. Vlaeyen JW, Linton SJ. Fear-avoidance and its consequences in chronic musculoskeletal pain: a state of the art. Pain 2000;85(3):317–32.

23. Philips HC. Avoidance behaviour and its role in sustaining chronic pain. Behav Res Ther 1987;25(4):273–9.

24. Waddell G, Newton M, Henderson I, et al. A Fear-Avoidance Beliefs Questionnaire (FABQ) and the role of fear-avoidance beliefs in chronic low back pain and disability. Pain 1993;52(2):157–68.

25. Vlaeyen JWS, de Jong J, Geilen M, et al. Graded exposure in vivo for pain-related fear. In: Gatchel RJ, Turk DC, editors. Psychological approaches to pain management: a practitioner's handbook. 2nd edition. New York: The Guilford Press; 2002. p. 210–33.

26. Bortz WM. The disuse syndrome. West J Med 1984;141(5):691–4.

27. Fordyce WE. Behavioral methods for chronic pain and illness. St. Louis: Mosby Year Book, Inc.; 1976.

28. Vlaeyen JWS, de Jong J, Geilen M, et al. Graded exposure in vivo in the treatment of pain-related fear: a replicated single-case experimental design in four patients with chronic low back pain. Behav Res Ther 2001;39:151–66.

29. Vlaeyen JW, de Jong J, Geilen M, et al. The treatment of fear of movement/(re)-injury in chronic low back pain: further evidence on the effectiveness of exposure in vivo. Clin J Pain 2002;18(4):251–61.

30. Boersma K, Linton S, Overmeer T, et al. Lowering fear-avoidance and enhancing function through exposure in vivo. A multiple baseline study across six patients with back pain. Pain 2004;108(1–2):8–16.

31. Jensen MP, Turner JA, Romano JM. Changes in beliefs, catastrophizing and coping are associated with improvement in multidisciplinary pain treatment. J Consult Clin Psychol 2001;69:655–62.

32. Boothby JL, Thorn BE, Stroud MW, et al. Coping with pain. In: Gatchel RJ, Turk DC, editors. Psychosocial factors in pain. New York: The Guilford Press; 1999. p. 343–59.

33. Jensen MP, Turner JA, Romano JM, et al. Coping with chronic pain: a critical review of the literature. Pain 1991;47(3):249–83.

34. Jensen MP, Turner JA, Romano JM, et al. Relationship of pain-specific beliefs to chronic pain adjustment. Pain 1994;57:301–9.

35. Turner JA, Jensen MP, Romano JM. Do beliefs, coping, and catastrophizing independently predict functioning in patients with chronic pain? Pain 2000;85(1–2): 115–25.

36. Tan G, Jensen MP, Robinson-Whelen S, et al. Coping with chronic pain: a comparison of two measures. Pain 2001;90(1–2):127–33.

37. Ramírez-Maestre C, Esteve R, López AE. Cognitive appraisal and coping in chronic pain patients. Eur J Pain 2008;12(6):749–56.
38. Jensen MP, Ehde DM, Hoffman AJ, et al. Cognitions, coping and social environment predict adjustment to phantom limb pain. Pain 2002;95(1–2):133–42.
39. Steultjens MP, Dekker J, Bijlsma JW. Coping, pain, and disability in osteoarthritis: a longitudinal study. J Rheumatol 2001;28(5):1068–72.
40. van Lankveld W, Van't PBP, van de Putte L, et al. Disease-specific stressors in rheumatoid arthritis: coping and well-being. Br J Rheumatol 1994;33(11):1067–73.
41. Nielson WR, Jensen MP, Hill ML. An activity pacing subscale for the chronic pain coping inventory: development in a sample of patients with fibromyalgia syndrome. Pain 2001;89:111–5.
42. Keefe FJ, Brown GK, Wallston KA, et al. Coping with rheumatoid arthritis pain: catastrophizing as a maladaptive strategy. Pain 1989;37(1):51–6.
43. Roth RS, Lowery JC, Hamill JB. Assessing persistent pain and its relation to affective distress, depressive symptoms, and pain catastrophizing in patients with chronic wounds: a pilot study. Am J Phys Med Rehabil 2004;83(11):827–34.
44. Cook AJ, Brawer PA, Vowles KE. The fear-avoidance model of chronic pain: validation and age analysis using structural equation modeling. Pain 2006;121: 195–206.
45. Demmelmaier I, Lindberg P, Åsenlöf P, et al. The associations between pain intensity, psychosocial variables, and pain duration/recurrence in a large sample of persons with nonspecific spinal pain. Clin J Pain 2008;24(7):611–9.
46. Jacobsen PB, Butler RW. Relation of cognitive coping and catastrophizing to acute pain and analgesic use following breast cancer surgery. J Behav Med 1996;19(1):17–29.
47. Sullivan MJ, Thorn B, Haythornthwaite JA, et al. Theoretical perspectives on the relation between catastrophizing and pain. Clin J Pain 2001;17(1):52–64.
48. Keefe FJ, Lefebvre JC, Egert JR, et al. The relationship of gender to pain, pain behavior, and disability in osteoarthritis patients: the role of catastrophizing. Pain 2000;87(3):325–34.
49. Turner JA, Jensen MP, Warms CA, et al. Catastrophizing is associated with pain intensity, psychological distress, and pain-related disability among individuals with chronic pain after spinal cord injury. Pain 2002;98(1–2):127–34.
50. Richardson C, Glenn S, Horgan M, et al. A prospective study of factors associated with the presence of phantom limb pain six months after major lower limb amputation in patients with peripheral vascular disease. J Pain 2007;8(10): 793–801.
51. Lee EJ, Wu MY, Lee GK, et al. Catastrophizing as a cognitive vulnerability factor related to depression in workers' compensation patients with chronic musculoskeletal pain. J Clin Psychol Med Settings 2008;15(3):182–92.
52. Sullivan MJ, D'Eon JL. Relation between catastrophizing and depression in chronic pain patients. J Abnorm Psychol 1990;99(3):260–3.
53. Geisser ME, Robinson ME, Keefe FJ, et al. Catastrophizing, depression and the sensory, affective and evaluative aspects of chronic pain. Pain 1994;59(1):79–83.
54. Ehde D, Jensen MP. Feasibility of a cognitive restructuring intervention for treatment of chronic pain in persons with disabilities. Rehabil Psychol 2004;49: 116–37.
55. Romano JM, Turner JA. Chronic pain and depression: does the evidence support a relationship? Psychol Bull 1985;97(1):18–34.
56. Bair MJ, Robinson RL, Katon W, et al. Depression and pain comorbidity: a literature review. Arch Intern Med 2003;163(20):2433–45.

57. Banks SM, Kerns RD. Explaining high rates of depression in chronic pain: a diathesis -stress framework. Psychol Bull 1996;119:95–110.
58. Alschuler KN, Theisen-Goodvich ME, Haig A. A comparison of the relationship between depression, perceived disability, and physical performance in persons with chronic pain. Eur J Pain 2008;12(6):757–64.
59. Gatchel RJ, Dersh J. Psychological disorders and chronic pain: are there cause-and-effect relationships? In: Turk DC, Gatchel RJ, editors. Psychological approaches to pain management: a practitioner's handbook. 2nd edition. New York: The Guilford Press; 2002. p. 30–51.
60. Fishbain DA, Cutler R, Rosomoff HL, et al. Chronic pain-associated depression: antecedent or consequence of chronic pain? A review. Clin J Pain 1997;13(2): 116–37.
61. Anderson RJ, Freedland KE, Clouse RE, et al. The prevalence of comorbid depression in adults with diabetes. Diabetes Care 2001;24:1069–78.
62. Robinson ME, Riley JL III. The role of emotion in pain. In: Gatchel RJ, Turk DC, editors. Psychosocial factors in pain. New York: The Guilford Press; 1999. p. 74–88.
63. Mok LC. Anxiety, depression and pain intensity in patients with low back pain who are admitted to acute care hospitals. J Clin Nurs 2008;17(11):1471–80.
64. Currie SR, Wang J. More data on major depression as an antecedent risk factor for first onset of chronic back pain. Psychol Med 2005;35(9):1275–82.
65. Linton SJ. A review of psychological risk factors in back and neck pain. Spine 2000;25(9):1148–56.
66. Maxwell TD, Gatchel RJ, Mayer TG. Cognitive predictors of depression in chronic low back pain: toward an inclusive model. J Behav Med 1998;21:131–43.
67. Smith TW, Peck JR, Milano RA, et al. Cognitive distortion in rheumatoid arthritis: relation to depression and disability. J Consult Clin Psychol 1988;56(3):412–6.
68. Smith TW, Christensen AJ, Peck JR, et al. Cognitive distortion, helplessness, and depressed mood in rheumatoid arthritis: a four-year longitudinal analysis. Health Psychol 1994;13(3):213–7.
69. Campbell LC, Clauw DJ, Keefe FJ. Persistent pain and depression: a biopsychosocial perspective. Biol Psychiatry 2003;54(3):399–409.
70. Rudy TE, Kerns RD, Turk DC. Chronic pain and depression: toward a cognitive-behavioral mediation model. Pain 1988;35(2):129–40.
71. Arnstein P, Caudill M, Mandle CL, et al. Self efficacy as a mediator of the relationship between pain intensity, disability, and depression in chronic pain patients. Pain 1999;80:483–91.
72. López-Martínez AE, Esteve-Zarazaga R, Ramírez-Maestre C. Perceived social support and coping responses are independent variables explaining pain adjustment among chronic pain patients. J Pain 2008;9(4):373–9.
73. Romano JM, Turner JA, Jensen MP. The family environment in chronic pain patients: comparison to controls and relationship to patient depression, disability, and pain behaviors. J Clin Psychol Med Settings 1997;4:383–95.
74. Skinner BF. Operant behavior. In: Honig WK, editor. Operant behavior: areas of research and application. New York: Appleton-Century-Crofts; 1966. p. 13–32.
75. Turk DC, Gatchel RJ. Psychosocial factors and pain: revolution and evolution. In: Gatchel RJ, Turk DC, editors. Psychosocial factors in pain: critical perspectives. New York: The Guilford Press; 1999. p. 481–93.
76. Fordyce WE, Fowler RS, Lehmann JF, et al. Some implications of learning in problems of chronic pain. J Chronic Dis 1968;21(3):179–90.
77. Romano JM, Turner JA, Jensen MP, et al. Chronic pain patient-spouse behavioral interactions predict patient disability. Pain 1995;63(3):353–60.

78. Romano JM, Turner JA, Friedman LS, et al. Sequential analysis of chronic pain behaviors and spouse responses. J Consult Clin Psychol 1992;60(5):777–82.
79. Block AR, Kremer EF, Gaylor M. Behavioral treatment of chronic pain: the spouse as a discriminative cue for pain behavior. Pain 1980;9(2):243–52.
80. Flor H, Kerns RD, Turk DC. The role of spouse reinforcement, perceived pain, and activity levels of chronic pain patients. J Psychosom Res 1987;31(2):251–9.
81. Morley S, Eccleston C, Williams A. Systematic review and meta-analysis of randomized controlled trials of cognitive behaviour therapy and behaviour therapy for chronic pain in adults, excluding headache. Pain 1999;80(1–2):1–13.

Updates in Cardiac Rehabilitation

Jennifer Dorosz, MD[a,b,*]

KEYWORDS

- Cardiac rehabilitation • Exercise training
- Secondary prevention • Heart disease • Physical conditioning

In the treatment of coronary artery disease and heart failure, cardiac rehabilitation has not had as much appeal to clinicians as other medical and invasive strategies; however, it is as beneficial in decreasing mortality as other common treatments such as b-blockers, aspirin, and angiotensin-converting enzyme inhibitors.[1] In fact, in the early twentieth century patients were prescribed months of bed rest after a myocardial infarction with the theory that inactivity would prevent mechanical complications. It was thought that extended bed rest was necessary for adequate wound healing, as the first pathologic studies of myocardial infarction showed that the time to scar formation from the initial insult was a prolonged 6-week process. Often patients never returned to work, and they were not allowed to participate in activities that required even a modest amount of physical effort, such as stair climbing.[2] It was not until the 1960s that increasing hospital costs prompted investigations into early mobilization and discharge. Subsequently a few supervised outpatient exercise programs were developed.[3] Studies done in the 1960s and 1970s proved that exercise for cardiac patients was safe, although no large long-term studies were powered to document a benefit until 1989, when meta-analysis showed that comprehensive cardiac rehabilitation and exercise training improved survival.[4] Today, exercise training in patients with a variety of cardiac diagnoses has been well studied and is an important part of secondary prevention. It is recommended in guideline statements by the American Heart Association, the American College of Cardiology, and the American Association of Cardiovascular and Pulmonary Rehabilitation, yet it is still underused.[5,6]

The purpose of this review is to discuss the benefits, clinical indications, safety, and specific protocols of cardiac rehabilitation. Most cardiac rehabilitation programs offer a combination of wellness counseling as well as a supervised exercise program. As advised by the Agency for Health Care Policy and Research and the National Institutes

[a] Division of Cardiology, University of Colorado, Aurora, CO, USA
[b] Cardiac & Vascular Center, Anschutz Inpatient Pavilion, 12605 E, 16th Avenue, Mail Stop B120, PO Box 6510, Aurora, CO 80045, USA
* Cardiac & Vascular Center, Anschutz Inpatient Pavilion, 12605 E, 16th Avenue, Mail Stop B120, PO Box 6510, Aurora, CO 80045.
E-mail address: jennifer.dorosz@uchsc.edu

Phys Med Rehabil Clin N Am 20 (2009) 719–736
doi:10.1016/j.pmr.2009.06.006
1047-9651/09/$ – see front matter © 2009 Elsevier Inc. All rights reserved.

of Health, a comprehensive education component should include advice on smoking cessation, diet and nutrition, weight loss, stress management, diabetes control, blood pressure reduction, and lipid management.[7] Although all these interventions are an important part of secondary prevention, this review focuses on the specific clinical benefits, physiologic effects, and methods of exercise training.

CLINICAL AND PHYSIOLOGIC BENEFITS

Numerous small studies have demonstrated that a supervised exercise program for patients with a variety of cardiac diagnoses improves quality of life, decreases the rate of reinfarction, reduces rehospitalization, and prevents ischemia.[8–13] In 1989 a meta-analysis of several randomized studies also showed a significant decrease in mortality of myocardial infarction survivors who participated in a comprehensive cardiac rehabilitation program compared with controls. The odds ratios for 1-, 2-, and 3-year survival were 0.77, 0.74, and 0.80, respectively.[4] Although this landmark study was done before the advent of current medical and invasive therapies now used to treat myocardial infarctions, a more recent study also found that cardiac rehabilitation had a similar effect on mortality in heart attack survivors.[14] In fact, the degree of benefit continued to increase in recent years, as those patients who participated in cardiac rehabilitation in 1998 fared better than controls compared with those who participated in 1982.[14] The most recent meta-analysis, consisting of 7683 patients, showed a 31% relative risk reduction in mortality for those who participated in an exercise-only form of cardiac rehabilitation.[15] Based on this analysis, 72 patients would have to participate in an exercise training program to save one life over 2.5 years.[16]

Exercise training improves outcomes and mortality in cardiac patients through a host of mechanisms. By directly measuring coronary atherosclerosis, Kramsch and colleagues[17] showed that exercise causes a regression in plaque burden. This effect is likely achieved by improving several atherogenic clinical parameters, such as by correcting dyslipidemia, reducing blood pressure, increasing insulin sensitivity, reducing adiposity, decreasing vascular inflammation, and augmenting endothelial function.

Exercise improves lipid profiles by causing a modest increase in high-density lipoprotein (HDL) and a decrease in low-density lipoprotein (LDL). HDL, the so-called good cholesterol, is an LDL scavenger and high levels are important to decrease atherogenesis. Although diet alone has little effect on HDL, a low-fat diet in combination with moderate exercise increases HDL levels by up to 5% to 13%.[18] LDL is the bad cholesterol. It is directly atherosclerotic and a major component in vessel injury. A 10% reduction in LDL levels is seen with an exercise and diet combination.[19] Less is known about the effects of exercise on triglycerides. Most studies show little effect in those patients with baseline normal triglyceride levels. Among those with diabetes or high triglyceride levels, however, exercise does improve hypertriglyceremia.[20–22]

By increasing muscle mass and efficient glucose utilization, exercise training specifically lowers insulin resistance. In fact, low basal levels of insulin are seen in well-trained nondiabetic subjects, despite a high carbohydrate and caloric diet.[23] Exercise begins to lower insulin resistance after only one exercise session, although its effect wanes after as few as 3 days of inactivity.[23] Chronic conditioning leads to chronically low insulin levels, signifying high insulin sensitivity. This effect is independent of body weight, percentage of body fat, and caloric intake.[24] In diabetics especially, decreasing insulin resistance has important clinical consequences. For example, 22 weeks of aerobic exercise training in type 2 diabetics reduces hemoglobin A1c values by 0.51%. A further decrease of hemoglobin A1c by 0.46% is seen if aerobic exercise is combined with resistance training.[25] The effect is greater for those with a baseline A1c greater than 7.5%. In this group, an average decrease of more than 1% was demonstrated without changing diet or medications.[25]

In hypertensive patients, exercise has an acute effect on blood pressure. Mean blood pressure is reduced an average of 7 mm Hg on days when patients participate in 30 minutes of moderate exercise.[26] Long-term exercise training has a sustained effect on blood pressure. After 32 weeks of supervised training in severely hypertensive patients, mean blood pressure was reduced by 5 mm Hg and allowed for a reduction in blood pressure medications.[27] These patients also demonstrated beneficial cardiac reverse remodeling on echo, showing a reduction in left ventricular hypertrophy and left ventricular mass.[27]

Improvements in atherogenic indices such as dyslipidemia, insulin resistance, and hypertension are seen despite only a small change in body mass index. In studies of weight loss during supervised exercise programs, the results are mixed.[28,29] Although there is likely a small decrease in weight (around 2 kg) with exercise alone,[29] obese patients must combine intensive diet with a moderate exercise program to achieve a more reasonable 8.5 kg weight loss or a 1.3 kg/m^2 drop in body mass index.[28,30]

In addition to contributing to a direct decrease in atherogenesis, exercise training may also have antithrombotic effects. There are increased serum levels of fibrinogen, a coagulant, after a myocardial infarction. Among survivors of a heart attack, this increased fibrinogen level is associated with additional events.[31] Fibrinolysis is mediated by tissue-type plasminogen activator (t-PA) and inhibited by plasminogen activator inhibitor type 1 (PAI-1). The activity of t-PA is increased in older men after a 6-week program of moderate exercise. This result is accompanied by a decrease in t-PA antibodies, PAI-1, and fibrinogen.[32] In contrast, platelet activation may actually increase temporarily in sedentary individuals who undergo strenuous exercise acutely, increasing their short-term risk of an event.[33] Long-term conditioning, however, mitigates the risk and leads to a chronic decrease in platelet activity and clot formation.[34]

Conditioning also has important anti-inflammatory effects. Markers of inflammation are higher in patients with coronary artery disease. Abnormal levels of highly sensitive C-reactive protein (hsCRP), tumor necrosis factor-α (TNF-α), and interleukin-6 (IL-6) have all correlated with an increased risk of future events.[35] In several studies, exercise training has been shown to decrease the levels of all these markers of vascular inflammation independent of weight loss, lipid management, or blood pressure.[36] In one study, patients with obstructive coronary artery disease were randomized to 2 years of exercise training without invasive intervention or percutaneous revascularization. Those in the exercise group decreased their hsCRP and IL-6 levels by 41% and 18%, respectively compared with no improvement in the stented group. Furthermore, the exercise group had fewer cardiovascular events and showed a greater improvement in exercise tolerance and ischemic threshold compared with the angioplasty group.[37]

A decrease in vascular inflammation, blood pressure, and LDL may contribute to better endothelial function, but there is also evidence that exercise training independently improves vascular function by promoting vasodilatation.[38] Arterial dilatation is mediated by endothelial release of nitric oxide which is impaired in atherosclerotic vessels, leading to a decrease in arterial area and blood flow.[39] Exercise training attenuates this effect. Indeed, a 4-week exercise program has shown to reduce the abnormal acetylcholine-induced vasoconstriction in diseased coronary arteries. Compared with the control group, the trained group also had an increase in coronary blood flow reserve by demonstrating a more vigorous response to vasodilators.[40]

Other evidence has shown that exercise training in diabetics improves vascular function better than pharmacologic therapy.[41] In patients with coronary artery disease, exercise has a direct positive effect on brachial artery reactivity and nitric oxide levels.[42]

In part through its effects on endothelial function, exercise training reduces ischemia and increases the ischemic threshold in patients with obstructive coronary artery disease. The combination of increased blood flow with more efficient cardiac metabolic capacity can decrease ischemic episodes despite an increase in workload.[43] Patients with chronic angina and documented ST depressions who participated in regular moderate exercise for 6 months were able to exercise longer and at higher workloads at the end of the training period.[44] They were able also to generate a higher heart rate, blood pressure, and myocardial oxygen demand before the onset of chest pain or electrocardiographic signs of ischemia.[45] More intense exercise training, with sessions that actually induce ischemia, is safe[46] and leads to increase coronary blood flow by promoting collateral formation.[47–50]

Physical conditioning also has a distinct antiarrhythmic effect, reducing the risk of sudden death. This effect is particularly important in patients with coronary artery disease or cardiomyopathies who have up to a 10% chance of developing fatal ventricular tachycardias or fibrillation within 1 year.[51] In animals susceptible to sudden death, exercise training significantly reduces the risk of developing a ventricular arrhythmia during electrophysiology testing.[52] This reduction in arrhythmic potential is in part mediated by altering the automatic nervous system. Patients with heart disease who have a high sympathetic tone are at increased risk of sudden death, and exercise helps mitigate this risk by lowering sympathetic activity while increasing parasympathetic activity.[53] Exercise training has been shown to lower resting heart rates, increase heart rate variability, and increase serum acetylcholine levels, all of which are associated with enhanced vagal tone and lower risk of sudden death.[53,54] There is also evidence that physical training has a direct effect on cardiac myocytes. Similar to β-blocker therapy, exercise reduces the abnormally high level of β2-adrenoceptor responsiveness seen in cardiac tissue after a myocardial infarct.[55,56] Exercise has also been shown to lengthen the refractory period of ventricular tissue, increasing electrical stability.[57] Thus, some investigators advocate that the decrease in mortality seen with cardiac rehabilitation may be entirely due to a reduction in arrhythmias leading to sudden death.[58]

Through a variety of mechanisms, the exercise-training portion of cardiac rehabilitation has many clinical and physiologic benefits that directly prolong life in cardiac patients. Some benefits, such as a reduction in LDL levels, hemoglobin A1c, blood pressure, and body mass index, can be easily measured and have a direct effect on reducing coronary atheromas. Other physiologic benefits, such as a reduction in thrombosis, inflammation, poor endothelial function, ischemia, and arrhythmias, may be harder to quantify but also play a role in improving health and survival.

INDICATIONS, CONTRAINDICATIONS, AND SAFETY

Exercise training is safe and effective for a variety of patient populations. Traditional indications for cardiac rehabilitation include patients recovering from a myocardial infarction or coronary artery bypass surgery; however, in 1995 a guideline statement jointly issued by the Agency for Health Care Policy and Research and the National Institutes of Health broadened the indications to include patients with stable angina and congestive heart failure.[59] In March of 2006, the Centers of Medicare and Medicaid issued a memorandum expanding coverage to patients who have had valve surgery or cardiac transplant.[60] **Table 1** lists the indications reimbursed by Medicare and the research studies cited to include each group. Despite clear evidence supporting exercise training in patients with nonischemic congestive heart failure,[67-70] the committee did not expand coverage for a diagnosis of heart failure alone.[60] As the Centers for Medicare and Medicaid usually sets the standards of coverage for the health insurance industry as a whole, most people outside the groups listed in **Table 1** are not covered. Some insurers, however, have recognized the clinical benefits and cost-effectiveness of cardiac rehabilitation and have agreed to cover other patient populations, including those with heart failure, peripheral artery disease, congenital heart disease, left ventricular assist devices, valvular disease, pacemakers, pulmonary hypertension, and cardiac arrhythmias.

To determine an individual's risk of starting an exercise program, a 4-category risk assessment has been proposed:[5]

Class A: Men younger than 45 years of age or women younger than 55 years with no known cardiac problems and no cardiovascular symptoms, or older individuals with no known symptoms and normal exercise tolerance demonstrated by stress testing

Class B: Those with known coronary artery disease, valve disease, congenital heart disease, or heart failure with stable New York Heart Association Class 1 or 2 symptoms

Class C: Patients with known coronary artery disease, valve disease, congenital heart disease, or heart failure with stable New York Heart Association Class 3 or 4 symptoms, evidence of ischemia at a low workload (less than 6 metabolic equivalents [METs]), a drop in blood pressure, or nonsustained ventricular tachycardia with exercise

Class D: Patients with known cardiovascular disease with unstable symptoms or angina, severe and symptomatic valvular disease, uncontrolled arrhythmias, or those with congenital heart disease for which there is a contraindication for exercise (like hypertrophic cardiomyopathy).

Supervised exercise training is designed for patients in classes B and C. Initially electrocardiography (EKG) and blood pressure monitoring should be performed during exercise sessions for those in class C. Individuals in class A can likely start

Table 1
Groups covered by Medicare for cardiac rehabilitation and associated trials cited by the centers for Medicare and Medicaid services

Eligible Criteria	Evidence to Support Coverage
Acute myocardial infarction in the last 12 months	Witt et al (2004)[14] Blumenthal et al (2005)[12]
Coronary artery bypass surgery	Hedback et al (2001)[61]
Stable angina	Agency for Healthcare Research and Quality (AHRQ)[62]
Valve repair or replacement	Stewart et al (2003)[63]
Percutaneous transluminal coronary angioplasty or coronary stenting	Stewart et al (2003)[63] Belardinelli et al (2001)[64] Dendale et al (2005)[13]
Heart or heart-lung transplant	Kavanagh et al (2005)[65] Hummel et al (2001)[66]

an exercise program without supervision. Those in class D should not exercise until further medical care can stabilize their symptoms and lower their risk.

Using this classification, supervised exercise training is very safe even in those with significant cardiovascular disease. The likelihood of a major event such as a cardiac arrest or myocardial infarction is less than 1 per 67,126 patient-hours of exercise.[71] Less severe complications (the development of chest pain, shortness of breath, or non–life-threatening arrhythmias which cause termination of the exercise session) occur at a rate of 1 per 320 hours.[72] The rate of death is about 1 per 783,972 patient-hours.[73] This mortality risk compares favorably to the rate of death in a control population of healthy joggers (1 per 396,000 hours).[74] Indeed, at 1 mortal event per approximately 80 exercise years, dying during a supervised exercise session may even be attributed to chance alone. The small rate of major complications has led some investigators to advocate that the current risk classification system is too strict.[1] Perhaps more patients should be allowed to exercise without monitoring, thus allowing for the establishment of more off-site, low-cost, and convenient exercise facilities.

EXERCISE PROTOCOLS

There are 3 sequential phases of cardiac rehabilitation.[75] Phase 1 focuses on the inpatient setting, and includes early mobilization and walking with nursing or physical therapy support 24 to 48 hours after an acute event. Phase 2 is a supervised exercise and counseling program that usually starts 2 to 6 weeks after discharge from the hospital. Phase 3 focuses on maintaining fitness at home or in a private gym after completion of a cardiac rehabilitation program.

On referral to cardiac rehabilitation (phase 2), an exercise prescription should be individualized for each patient based on his or her medical diagnoses and baseline stamina. An initial history and physical should define medical conditions and identify those with unstable symptoms. It should also pinpoint each patient's modifiable risk factors, such as ongoing smoking or obesity, to customize the education programs.[76] A baseline symptom-limited exercise stress test is also recommended.[5] This test determines the patient's maximum exercise tolerance and heart rate in order to tailor future workouts. If ischemia (>1 mm of horizontal ST depression on EKG monitoring) or arrhythmias develop during exercise testing, this level of exercise and heart rate should be recorded. These patients warrant EKG and blood pressure monitoring during exercise. Future sessions should target a heart rate 10 to 15 beats below the ischemic threshold.[5] Patients with internal cardiac defibrillators should also have close monitoring of their heart rate during exercise testing and rehabilitation sessions. The heart rate should be kept below the set threshold that would trigger device therapy or shocks.

Exercise intensity can be determined in an individual by measuring the maximum oxygen uptake (Vo_{2max}). Vo_{2max} is defined as the maximum oxygen uptake that can be achieved in an individual with progressive exercise.[77] This value can be quantified using gas analyzers that measure the breath-by-breath concentration of oxygen and carbon dioxide. During standard exercise testing and cardiac rehabilitation, however, these sophisticated tests are not usually needed. Instead, exercise intensity is more often expressed in METs, which is defined as the uptake of oxygen for the average individual for a given activity. One MET is equal to a Vo_2 of 3.5 mL O_2/kg/min and is the amount of oxygen uptake for the average person at rest.[77] **Table 2** lists the average maximum exercise intensity by age and compares it with standard activities and METs.[5] An average sedentary man can achieve a maximum of 10 METs, whereas

Table 2			
Average maximum exercise tolerance for healthy sedentary adults by age			
Age	Vo_{2max}	METs	Example Activity
20–39	42 mL O_2/kg/min	12.0	Skipping rope
40–64	35 mL O_2/kg/min	10.0	Jogging at 6 miles (9.6 km)/h
65–79	28 mL O_2/kg/min	8.0	Walking at 3.5 miles (5.6 km)/h
>80	17.5 mL O_2/kg/min	5.0	Doubles tennis

many well-trained distance runners can reach up to 24 METs. The failure to achieve at least 6 METs in patients less than 80 years of age is a marker of severe deconditioning or disease and carries a poor prognosis.

Exercise intensity can also be measured by the rating of perceived exertion. On this Borg Scale, a patient rates his or her level of perceived work from 6 to 20.[78] A level of 12 to 13 is rated "somewhat hard" and generally corresponds to 60% of Vo_{2max}. A rating of 18, "very hard," corresponds to 85% of Vo_{2max}. This method of determining exercise intensity is particularly helpful in patients who are on high-dose b-blockers or in heart transplant patients, in whom the heart rate is a less reliable indicator of exertion level. Otherwise, the rating of perceived exertion, Vo_{2max}, maximum achieved METs, and maximum heart rate are closely correlated in most groups of cardiac patients.

During a supervised exercise program, patients typically meet for an exercise session 3 to 5 times a week. Each exercise session should begin with a 5- to 10-minute warm-up period during which they participate in light stretches. Sessions should then include 20 to 60 minutes of endurance aerobic activity. Another 5 to 10 minutes of cool-down with walking and stretching are important to prevent dizziness associated with the sudden cessation of moderate exercise. Most sessions (2–3 times a week) should also include resistance training with specific exercises to strengthen each muscle group.

The endurance portion of the session usually progresses in stages.[5] The first 4 to 6 weeks are focused on exercises with a light intensity level. Light intensity is defined as 20% to 40% of the maximum METs, a perceived exertion score of 10 to 11, or 35% to 55% of the maximum heart rate. During this time the participant may have limited endurance (20 minutes or less). Over the next 4 to 6 months the exercise sessions should progress to a moderate intensity level (40% to 60% of maximum METs, a perceived exertion score of 12 to 13, or 55% to 70% of maximum heart rate). During this time, the participant should also focus on endurance, gradually increasing the aerobic workout to 40 to 60 minutes. After 6 to 12 months, the goal is to maintain the achieved fitness level by continuing the program at home or in a private gym. Although a treadmill has been the traditional mode for endurance exercise testing and training in the United States, patients may prefer other modes of aerobic exercise such as elliptical machines, stair climbers, bicycling, or even swimming. During a cardiac rehabilitation session they may often switch between several of these modalities. Indeed, several 10-minute sessions are as beneficial as one longer session.[5]

Resistance and strength training are an important part of a cardiac rehabilitation program. Although it has little effect on Vo_{2max}, resistance training helps increase strength, basal metabolic rate, endurance time, and functional capacity, while reducing injuries. It is especially important in the frail and elderly.[79] Recommended exercises include the chest press, shoulder press, triceps extension, biceps curl, arm pull-down (for the upper back), low back extension, abdominal curl, quadriceps extension, hamstring curl, and calf raise. A prescription of one set of 10 to 15 repetitions with light weight (for a goal perceived exertion score of 10–11) for 8 of these exercises per session is recommended for patients with cardiac disease.[79] Patients who have had a sternotomy should avoid weight training with the upper extremities for 3 months after the operation, and stability of the sternum should be examined before starting upper-body weight lifting.[5] **Table 3** gives a sample workout schedule for a training session.

Ideally, 6 months of cardiac rehabilitation with 3 sessions a week is recommended.[5] Depending on a patient's progress and compliance, the number of sessions and time can vary between 6 weeks and 12 months. The Centers of Medicare and Medicaid Services generally recommends (and pays for) 36 sessions over 12 weeks; however, there is an option to increase the number of sessions to 72 over a 36-week period "at the discretion of the contractor."[60]

To receive proper reimbursement from Medicare and other insurance groups, the individual programs should meet the Medicare guidelines for a supervised cardiac rehabilitation training center.[60] These include the ability to perform heart rate monitoring as appropriate, provide supervision by staff trained in Advanced Cardiac Life Support, ensure proper recording of a patient's progress, symptoms, and complications, and allow for frequent communication with the primary or referring doctor. One costly requirement is that a cardiologist be on site during each exercise session, and that there is team in place to handle cardiac emergencies. There is some controversy on how best to meet these requirements. For centers located in an inpatient hospital, these responsibilities are assigned by a staff cardiologist or medical director working on the premises and a hospital code team. It is also recommended that the medical director also personally attend a patient's exercise session to assess progress at the beginning and middle of the course.[80] These requirements, however, may be infeasible or cost-prohibitive for facilities not connected to a hospital.

GOALS AND MEASURES OF SUCCESS

In addition to reducing mortality, cardiac risk factors, and future events, a major goal of cardiac rehabilitation is increasing a patient's functional capacity and, in elderly patients, reducing frailty. Indeed, after just 12 weeks of exercise training, patients are able to increase their maximum METs from an average of 6.6 to 8.7 (32%).[81] Other studies have also shown a similar increase in functional activity ranging from 36% to 50% in both men and women who complete a cardiac rehabilitation program. Severe coronary artery disease and congestive heart failure should not exclude one from

Table 3				
Sample workout schedule for cardiac rehabilitation sessions				
Exercise	Time (Minutes)	Goal METs (% of Maximum)	Goal Heart Rate (% of Maximum)	Borg Scale
Warm-up	5–10	Minimal		
Endurance exercise				
Initial period (0–6 weeks)	20	20%–40%	35%–55%	10–11
Final period (4–6 months)	40–60	40%–60%	55%–70%	12–13
Cool-down	5–10	Minimal		
Strength training	10–15 repetitions in 8 different exercises			10–11

participation in cardiac rehabilitation. In fact, there is a particularly high rate of improvement in those who begin with very low exercise tolerance (<5 METs). These subjects increased levels from an average of 4.1 to 8.3 METs.[82] Furthermore, patients who experience a large myocardial infarction (with creatine kinase levels >5000 U/L) achieve greater benefit in Vo_{2max} with exercise training than those with a small infarct.[83] Perhaps because of their improvement in fitness, patients who complete a 12-week exercise program report a substantial increase in quality of life. These patients have fewer physiologic symptoms associated with depression, anxiety, and somatization. They also report an increase in energy, a decrease in chronic pain, and overall better general health.[84]

Although they may begin with a significantly lower exercise tolerance, the elderly who participate in exercise training are not excluded from its benefits. Indeed, cardiac patients older than 75 years have as great or a greater increase in exercise tolerance than younger patients.[82,85] These patients also show improvements in risk factors with a reduction in LDL cholesterol, hypertension, and body mass index while reporting a similar increase in general well-being and overall quality of life compared with a younger cohort.[85] In fact, the elderly who maintain even modest levels of physical activity (like walking) live longer with less morbidity.[86] As with endurance training, the elderly should not be excluded from strength training. Weight lifting is important in this group to increase lean muscle mass, decrease orthopedic overuse injuries and falls, and promote independent living by increasing the ability to undertake routine activities.[79] Some older patients may have specific limitations with certain exercises due to arthritis and other comorbidities, so they may prefer more variety in their exercise sessions. In general, however, they can follow the same exercise prescription noted in the prior section.[5] Despite a psychosocial bias against exercise in the elderly, they certainly should not be excluded from cardiac rehabilitation programs.[87]

For those patients who were working before their cardiac event, a return to work is an important goal of exercise training. At present, only about 65% of patients who were working before a heart attack return to the workforce.[88] There is a need for more research on how cardiac rehabilitation can improve return-to-work rates. Despite clear evidence that exercise training increases physical conditioning, there are few studies proving that it also facilitates reemployment.[89,90] Rather, the rate of return to work may be more related to the specific social and economic situation of each patient, with a higher rate of reemployment among professionals and those ineligible for disability or other benefits.[89] In addition, individuals at low risk (patients less than 75 years, ejection fraction of >45%, absence of sustained ventricular arrhythmias, and the ability to achieve at least 7 METs on an exercise test without ischemic EKG changes) should be able to safely return to work and all usual activities within 2 weeks of hospital discharge; cardiac rehabilitation may not offer additional economic benefits regarding return to work.[91] However, there is a role for exercise training in those at higher risk or with a lower baseline functional ability, especially in those patients with heart failure, cardiomyopathy, or post-bypass surgery.[92,93] These patients benefit from the increase in exercise tolerance and sense of well-being associated with cardiac rehabilitation that may allow them to return to work in higher numbers. There is a personal and societal benefit in promoting a quick return to work, rather than have patients rely on disability. To that end, some exercise programs have been developed with this specific goal in mind. One German study showed that verbally setting a goal to return to work with both the patient and trainers has increased the percentage of patients who resumed their jobs.[94] Another study showed that tailoring an exercise program to a patient's pre-illness occupation, with specific work simulation, results in a substantial rate of reemployment in the same job.[95]

Thus, there may be a role for adjusting the type and goals of rehabilitation for preretirement patients to promote continued employment after a cardiac event.

COST-EFFECTIVENESS

In 1994, about 14% of the total United States health care budget was spent on the treatment of cardiac disease, amounting to about $130 billion.[96] These costs have likely already increased and will continue to increase as the prevalence of cardiac diseases continues to escalate in a population of increasing age and risk factors. Furthermore, many of the current treatments such as stenting, surgery, and defibrillators are invasive and cost-intensive. Because it may be as effective, cardiac rehabilitation offers cheap adjunctive therapy for cardiac patients.

Although the cost-effectiveness of cardiac rehabilitation has only been studied in a few older trials, it is clear that it saves money in reducing future hospitalizations, promoting reemployment, increasing quality of life, and decreasing mortality.[97–100] Oldridge and colleagues[99] evaluated a small group of patients after admission for acute myocardial infarction and found that the cost of rehabilitation per quality-adjusted life saved in 1991 US dollars was $9200. This amount was far cheaper than many other common cardiac treatments at the time, such as single-vessel bypass surgery ($68,000), treatment of hypertension with captopril ($106,900), or treatment of cholesterol with lovastatin ($17,000).[99] This study estimated the mean direct costs of an 8-week-long cardiac rehabilitation program to be around $790. This price included the cost of equipment and personnel to the rehabilitation center and the costs of transportation to the patient. There was also a saving of $310 in future outpatient consultations and medication reductions.[99] Because of their small patient group and short follow-up time, Oldridge and colleagues did not find a significant cost saving in future hospitalizations. Others, however, have shown that those who complete a 36-week program save an average of $900 (in 1997 US dollars) in 3-year hospital admission costs, almost making up the cost of the rehabilitation program itself ($1152) without considering other variables such as reduced mortality, medication reduction, and return to work.[100] In this study the estimated cost per life saved was $4950 (US, 1997).[100] These results are supported by a Swedish study in 1991 in which the costs of a cardiac rehabilitation program were outweighed by the savings from reduced hospitalizations and increased productivity of heart attack survivors, saving the Swedish health care system $12,000 (US, 1991) per enrolled patient over 5 years.[98] For patients, private insurance companies, Medicare, and society, cardiac rehabilitation is one of the most cost-effective options in the treatment of cardiac patients.

UNDERUSE

Despite its proven benefits and cost-effectiveness, cardiac rehabilitation is highly underused. A recent study identified more than 260,000 Medicare patients eligible for cardiac rehabilitation by surviving coronary bypass surgery or a myocardial infarction in 1997.[101] In that year, only 13% of the heart attack patients and 31% of the bypass patients (18% of the total) participated in at least one session of cardiac rehabilitation. Other studies done on a broader spectrum of patients of varying ages and insurance coverage confirm similarly low levels of enrollment.[102] Women, the elderly, nonwhites, the poor, and uninsured are disproportionately underrepresented in rehabilitation programs.[101,103]

A significant factor contributing to low participation rates is the failure of physicians to refer patients to cardiac rehabilitation programs. Ideally, most patients would be referred at hospital discharge,[76] otherwise the order should be written at the first follow-up visit. One study showed that only 8.7% of eligible patients at a university hospital were referred to rehabilitation. The elderly were far less likely to be referred, with a 3% decline in referral rates for each year of advanced age.[104] The uninsured were almost 3 times less likely to be referred.[104] There is also a strong bias against referring women, particularly older women, to exercise training.[105] Yet these underserved groups are as likely to benefit from exercise training as young men.[105] Furthermore, a strong recommendation from a patient's primary provider is the most powerful predictor of a patient's willingness to participate in a rehabilitation program.[106] In an effort to combat these low referral rates and biases, a joint guideline statement from the American Association of Cardiovascular and Pulmonary Rehabilitation, the American Heart Association, and the American College of Cardiology was recently issued. It emphasizes increased awareness of the benefits of cardiac rehabilitation, the implementation of automatic referral forms for both hospitalized and ambulatory patients, systematic data collection of referral rates and patterns, and ongoing performance measures for every hospital.[76]

There are also significant patient-related factors that prevent participation in rehabilitation services. Up to 50% of referred patients fail to enroll in rehabilitation services.[107] Not surprisingly, patients who live further away from an available rehabilitation program participate at lower rates. For example, those who live more than 15 miles from the nearest facility were 71% less likely to enroll than those who live within 1.5 miles.[101] There is also a large variation in enrollment rates between states. Idaho has a 6.6% participation rate whereas Nebraska has a 54% participation rate. Those states with the highest participation have more facilities per capita, and some have instituted a computerized system to order referrals and identify the nearest facility for each patient.[101]

Many providers have advocated in-home rehabilitation as a way to lower costs and expand coverage.[1] Typically these programs allow for 3 to 4 home visits by nurses or physical therapists who design an exercise program and monitor each patient's progress. Among low-risk patients, these programs have been shown to be as safe and effective as hospital-based, monitored training sessions.[108–110] However, for those at higher risk, particularly heart failure patients, these programs have failed to show equal efficacy and have higher event rates.[111]

An increase in the number of facilities, particularly in rural or underserved areas, is also needed; however, there is little enthusiasm for allocating resources to build and staff such programs. In 2006, when the Centers for Medicare Services reevaluated cardiac rehabilitation, it increased the reimbursement rate to $34 per session,[60] yet many argue that this reimbursement rate is too low to cover the costs. Compared with other cardiac procedures and interventions, cardiac rehabilitation does not allow for substantial revenue generation, discouraging organizations to expand these services.

A combination of interventions is needed to increase participation in this valuable service, including increased education of physicians and patients, a societal commitment to raise funding and reimbursement, the implementation of automatic referral programs, and the expansion in the numbers and types of available programs.

SUMMARY

Cardiac rehabilitation is an integral part of secondary prevention in those patients with a host of cardiac diagnosis. In particular, exercise training lowers blood pressure, improves cholesterol parameters, facilitates weight loss, reduces ischemia, and lowers insulin resistance. It also directly affects myocyte and endothelial function by lowing inflammation, increasing coronary blood flow, decreasing clot formation, and reducing arrhythmias. Through these mechanisms exercise training directly leads to better quality of life, physical conditioning, and survival of participating patients. Although rehabilitation does require a long-term commitment, exercise training protocols are simple, noninvasive, and safe. Compared with other common treatments for cardiac disease it is more effective and cheaper. It is directly cost-effective, saving costs for both society and the individual patient in future hospitalizations, doctor visits, and medication use, and loss of employment. Unfortunately, cardiac rehabilitation is highly underused as only a small proportion of eligible patients are referred to exercise programs, and fewer still complete a full course. Methods to improve referral patterns and compliance, especially among certain disadvantaged groups, should be explored.

REFERENCES

1. Bairey Merz CN, Paul-Labrador M, Vongvanich P. Time to reevaluate risk stratification guidelines for medically supervised exercise training in patients with coronary artery disease. JAMA 2000;283(11):1476–8.
2. Pashkow FJ. Issues in contemporary cardiac rehabilitation. J Am Coll Cardiol 1993;21(3):822–34.
3. Hellerstein HK, Hirsch EZ, Cumbler W, et al. Reconditioning of the coronary patient—a preliminary report. In: Likoff W, Moyer J, editors. Coronary heart disease. New York: Grune & Stratton; 1963. p. 447.
4. O'Connor GT, Buring JE, Yusuf S, et al. An overview of randomized trials of rehabilitation with exercise after myocardial infarction. Circulation 1989;80(2):234–44.
5. Fletcher GF, Balady GJ, Amsterdam EA, et al. Exercise standards for testing and training: a statement for healthcare professionals from the American Heart Association. Circulation 2001;104(14):1694–740.
6. Balady GJ, Williams MA, Ades PA, et al. Core components of cardiac rehabilitation/secondary prevention programs: 2007 update: a scientific statement from the American Heart Association: Exercise, Cardiac Rehabilitation, and Prevention Committee; the Council on Clinical Cardiology; the Councils on Cardiovascular Nursing, Epidemiology and Prevention, and Nutrition, Physical Activity, and Metabolism; and the American Association of Cardiovascular and Pulmonary Rehabilitation. Circulation 2007;115:2675–82.
7. Ades P. Cardiac rehabilitation and secondary prevention of coronary heart disease. N Engl J Med 2001;345:892–902.
8. Wilhelmsen L, Sanne H, Elmfeldt D, et al. A controlled trial of physical training after myocardial infarction: effects on risk factors, nonfatal reinfarction, and death. Prev Med 1975;4:491–508.
9. Vermeulen A, Lie KI, Durrer D. Effects of cardiac rehabilitation after myocardial infarction: changes in coronary risk factors and long-term prognosis. Am Heart J 1983;105(5):798–801.
10. Froelicher V, Jensen D, Genter F, et al. A randomized trial of exercise training in patients with coronary heart disease. JAMA 1984;252:1291–7.
11. Shaw LW, Oberman A, Barnes G, et al. Effects of a prescribed supervised exercise program on mortality and cardiovascular morbidity in patients after a myocardial infarction: the national exercise and heart disease project. Am J Cardiol 1981;48:39–46.

12. Blumenthal J, Sherwood A, Babyak M, et al. Effects of exercise and stress management training on markers of cardiovascular risk in patients with ischemic heart disease: a randomized controlled trial. JAMA 2005;293:1626–34.

13. Dendale P, Berger J, Hansen D, et al. Cardiac rehabilitation reduces the rate of major adverse cardiac events after percutaneous coronary intervention. Eur J Cardiovasc Nurs 2005;4:113–6.

14. Witt B, Jacobsen S, Weston S, et al. Cardiac rehabilitation after myocardial infarction in the community. J Am Coll Cardiol 2004;44:988–96.

15. Jolliffe JA, Rees K, Taylor RS, et al. Exercise-based rehabilitation for coronary heart disease. Cochrane Database Syst Rev 2001;1:CD001800.

16. Oldridge N, Perkins A, Marchionni N, et al. Number needed to treat in cardiac rehabilitation. J Cardiopulm Rehabil 2002;22(1):22–30.

17. Kramsch DM, Aspen AJ, Abramowitz BM, et al. Reduction of coronary atherosclerosis by moderate conditioning exercise in monkeys on an atherogenic diet. N Engl J Med 1981;305:1483–9.

18. Wood PD, Stefanick ML, Williams PT, et al. The effects on plasma lipoproteins of a prudent weight-reducing diet, with or without exercise, in overweight men and women. N Engl J Med 1991;325:461–6.

19. Stefanick ML, Mackey S, Sheehan M, et al. Effects of diet and exercise in men and postmenopausal women with low levels of HDL cholesterol and high levels of LDL cholesterol. N Engl J Med 1998;339:12–20.

20. Misra A, Alappan NK, Vikram NK, et al. Effect of supervised progressive resistance-exercise training protocol on insulin sensitivity, glycemia, lipids, and body composition in Asian Indians with type 2 diabetes. Diabetes Care 2008;7:1282–7.

21. Wagner H, Degerblad M, Thorell A, et al. Combined treatment with exercise training and acarbose improves metabolic control and cardiovascular risk factor profile in subjects with mild type 2 diabetes. Diabetes Care 2006;7:1471–7.

22. Sixt S, Rastan A, Desch S, et al. Exercise training but not rosiglitazone improves endothelial function in prediabetic patients with coronary disease. Eur J Cardiovasc Prev Rehabil 2008;15:473–8.

23. LeBlanc J, Nadeau A, Richard R, et al. Studies on the sparing effect of exercise on insulin requirements in human subjects. Metabolism 1981;30:1119–24.

24. Regensteiner JG, Shetterly SM, Meyer EJ, et al. Relationship between physical activity and insulin among persons with glucose intolerance: the San Luis Valley diabetes study. Diabetes Care 1995;18:490–7.

25. Sigal RJ, Kenny GP, Boule NG, et al. Effects of aerobic training, resistance training, or both on glycemic control in type 2 diabetes. Ann Intern Med 2007;147:357–9.

26. Pescatello LS, Fargo AE, Leach CN, et al. Short-term effect of dynamic exercise on arterial blood pressure. Circulation 1991;83:1557–61.

27. Kokkinos PF, Narayan P, Colleran JA, et al. Effects of regular exercise on blood pressure and left ventricular hypertrophy in African-American men with severe hypertension. N Engl J Med 1995;333:1462–7.

28. King AC, Tribble DL. The role of exercise in weight regulation in nonathletes. Sports Med 1991;11:331–49.

29. Pacy PJ, Webster J, Garrow JS. Exercise and obesity. Sports Med 1986;3:89–113.

30. Gondoni LA, Titon AM, Nibbio F, et al. Short-term effects of a hypocaloric diet and a physical activity programme on weight loss and exercise capacity in obese subjects with chronic ischaemic heart disease: a study in everyday practice. Acta Cardiol 2008;63(2):153–9.

31. Kannel WB, Wolf PA, Castelli WP, et al. Fibrinogen and risk of cardiovascular disease: the Framingham study. JAMA 1987;258:1183–6.
32. Stratton JR, Chandler WL, Schwartz RS, et al. Effects of physical conditioning on fibrinolytic variables and fibrinogen in young and old healthy adults. Circulation 1991;83:1692–7.
33. Kestin AS, Ellis PA, Barnard MR, et al. Effect of strenuous exercise on platelet activation state and reactivity. Circulation 1993;88:1502–11.
34. Gonzales F, Mañas M, Seiquer I, et al. Blood platelet function in healthy individuals of different ages: effects of exercise and exercise conditioning. J Sports Med Phys Fitness 1996;36:112–6.
35. Ridker PM, Hennekens CH, Buring JE, et al. C-reactive protein and other markers of inflammation in the prediction of cardiovascular disease in women. N Engl J Med 2000;342:836–43.
36. Walther C, Möbius-Winkler S, Linke A, et al. Regular exercise training compared with percutaneous intervention leads to a reduction of inflammatory markers and cardiovascular events in patients with coronary artery disease. Eur J Cardiovasc Prev Rehabil 2008;15:107–12.
37. Kim YJ, Shin YO, Bae JS, et al. Beneficial effects of cardiac rehabilitation and exercise after percutaneous coronary intervention on hsCRP and inflammatory cytokines in CAD patients. Pflugers Arch 2008;455:1081–8.
38. Green DJ, Walsh JH, Maiorana A, et al. Exercise-induced improvement in endothelial dysfunction is not mediated by changes in CV risk factors: pooled analysis of diverse patient populations. Am J Physiol Heart Circ Physiol 2003;24:1681–9.
39. Meredith IT, Yeung AC, Weidinger FF, et al. Role of impaired endothelium-dependent vasodilation in ischemic manifestations of coronary artery disease. Circulation 1993;87:V56–66.
40. Hambrecht R, Wolf A, Gielen S, et al. Effect of exercise on coronary endothelial function in patients with coronary artery disease. N Engl J Med 2000;342:454–60.
41. Maiorana A, O'Driscoll G, Cheetham C, et al. The effect of combined aerobic and resistance exercise training on vascular function in type 2 diabetes. J Am Coll Cardiol 2001;38:860–6.
42. Kingwell BA, Sherrard B, Jennings GL, et al. Four weeks of cycle training increases basal production of nitric oxide from the forearm. Am J Physiol 1997;272:H1070–7.
43. Squires RW. Mechanisms by which exercise training may improve the clinical status of cardiac patients. In: Schmidt DH, editor. Heart disease and rehabilitation. 3rd edition. Champaign (IL): Human Kinetics; 1995. p. 147–60.
44. Laslett LJ, Paumer L, Amsterdam EA. Increase in myocardial oxygen consumption indexes by exercise training at onset of ischemia in patients with coronary artery disease. Circulation 1985;71:958–62.
45. Ehsani AA, Heath GW, Hagberg JM, et al. Effects of 12 months of intense exercise training on ischemic ST-segment depression in patients with coronary artery disease. Circulation 1981;64:1116–24.
46. Noël M, Jobin J, Marcoux A, et al. Can prolonged exercise-induced myocardial ischaemia be innocuous? Eur Heart J 2007;28(13):1559–65.
47. Cohen MV, Yipintsoi T, Scheuer J. Coronary collateral stimulation by exercise in dogs with stenotic coronary arteries. J Appl Physiol 1982;52:664–71.
48. Lu X, Wu T, Huang P, et al. Effect and mechanism of intermittent myocardial ischemia induced by exercise on coronary collateral formation. Am J Phys Med Rehabil 2008;7(10):803–14.

49. Roth DM, White FC, Nichols ML, et al. Effect of long-term exercise on regional myocardial function and coronary collateral development after gradual coronary artery occlusion in pigs. Circulation 1990;82(5):1778–89.

50. Walsh JH, Bilsborough W, Maiorana A, et al. Exercise training improves conduit vessel function in patients with coronary artery disease. J Appl Physiol 2003;95: 20–5.

51. Buxton AE, Lee KL, Fisher JD, et al. A randomized study of the prevention of sudden death in patients with coronary artery disease. N Engl J Med 1999;341:1882–90.

52. Billman GE, Schwartz PJ, Stone HL. The effects of daily exercise on suscepti- bility to sudden cardiac death. Circulation 1984;69(6):1182–9.

53. DeSchryver C, Mertens-Strythaggen J. Heart tissue acetylcholine in chronically exercised rats. Experientia 1975;31:316–8.

54. Billman GE, Kukielka M. Effect of endurance exercise training on heart rate onset and heart rate recovery responses to submaximal exercise in animals suscep- tible to ventricular fibrillation. J Appl Physiol 2007;102(1):231–40.

55. Holycross BJ, Kukielka M, Nishijima Y, et al. Exercise training normalizes beta-adrenoceptor expression in dogs susceptible to ventricular fibrillation. Am J Physiol Heart Circ Physiol 2007;293(5):H2702–9.

56. Billman GE, Kukielka M, Kelley R, et al. Endurance exercise training attenuates cardiac beta2-adrenoceptor responsiveness and prevents ventricular fibrillation in animals susceptible to sudden death. Am J Physiol Heart Circ Physiol 2006; 290(6):H2590–9.

57. Such L, Alberola AM, Such-Miquel L, et al. Effects of chronic exercise on myocardial refractoriness: a study on isolated rabbit heart. Acta Physiol 2008; 193:331–9.

58. Billman GE. Aerobic exercise conditioning: a non-pharmacological antiar- rhythmic intervention. J Appl Physiol 2002;92:446–54.

59. Wenger NK, Froehlicher ES, Smith LK, et al. Cardiac rehabilitation clinical prac- tice guidelines. Rockville (MD): Agency for Health Care Policy and Research and the National Heart, Lung, and Blood Institute; 1995. (AHCPR publication No. 96-0672).

60. Phurrough SE, Salive M, Baldwin J, et al. Decision memo for cardiac rehabilita- tion programs (CAG-00089R). Centers for Medicare and Medicaid Services. Arlington (VA), March 22, 2006.

61. Hedback B, Perk J, Hornblad M, et al. Cardiac rehabilitation after coronary artery bypass surgery: 10-year results on mortality, morbidity and readmissions to hospital. J Cardiovasc Risk 2001;8:153–8.

62. Agency for Healthcare Research and Quality (AHRQ) Technology Assessment Program. Randomized trials of secondary prevention programs in coronary artery disease: a systematic review 2005. US Department of Health and Human Services. Rockville (MD).

63. Stewart K, Badenhop D, Brubaker P, et al. Cardiac rehabilitation following percu- taneous revascularization, heart transplant, heart valve surgery, and for chronic heart failure. Chest 2003;123:2104–11.

64. Belardinelli R, Paolini I, Cianci G, et al. Exercise training intervention after coronary angioplasty: the ETICA trial. J Am Coll Cardiol 2001;37(7):1891–900.

65. Kavanagh T, Mertens DJ, Shephard RJ, et al. Long-term cardiorespiratory results of exercise training following cardiac transplantation. Am J Cardiol 2003;91:190–4.

66. Hummel M, Michauk I, Hetzer R, et al. Quality of life after heart and heart-lung transplantation. Transplant Proc 2001;33:3546–8.

67. Jonsdottir S, Andersen K, Sigurosson A, et al. The effect of physical training in chronic heart failure. Eur J Heart Fail 2006;8(1):97–101.
68. Ko J, McKelvie R. The role of exercise training for patients with heart failure. Eura Medicophys 2005;41:35–47.
69. Rees K, Taylor RS, Singh S, et al. Exercise based rehabilitation for heart failure. Cochrane Database Syst Rev 2004;(3):CD003331.
70. Klecha A, Kawecka-Jaszcz K, Bacior B, et al. Physical training in patients with chronic heart failure of ischemic origin: effect on exercise capacity and left ventricular remodeling. Eur J Cardiovasc Prev Rehabil 2007;14(1):85–91.
71. Vongvanich P, Paul-Labrador MJ, Bairey Merz CN, et al. Safety of medically supervised exercise in a cardiac rehabilitation center. Am J Cardiol 1996; 77(15):1383–5.
72. Vongvanich P, Bairey Merz CN. Supervised exercise and electrocardiographic monitoring during cardiac rehabilitation. J Cardiopulm Rehabil 1996;16:233–8.
73. Van Camp SP, Peterson RA. Cardiovascular complications of outpatient cardiac rehabilitation programs. JAMA 1986;256:1160–3.
74. Thompson P, Funk E, Carleton R, et al. Incidence of death during jogging in Rhode Island from 1975 through 1980. JAMA 1982;247:2535–8.
75. Squires RW, Gau GT, Miller TD, et al. Cardiovascular rehabilitation: status 1990. Mayo Clin Proc 1990;65:731–55.
76. Thomas RJ, King M, Lui K, et al. AACVPR/ACC/AHA 2007 performance measures on cardiac rehabilitation for referral to and delivery of cardiac rehabilitation/secondary prevention services endorsed by the American College of Chest Physicians, American College of Sports Medicine, American Physical Therapy Association, Canadian Association of Cardiac Rehabilitation, European Association for Cardiovascular Prevention and Rehabilitation, InterAmerican Heart Foundation, National Association of Clinical Nurse Specialists, Preventive Cardiovascular Nurses Association, and the Society of Thoracic Surgeons. J Am Coll Cardiol 2007;50(14):1400–33.
77. Pollack ML, Wilmore JH. Exercise in health and disease: evaluation and prescription for prevention and rehabilitation. Philadelphia: Sauders; 1990.
78. Borg G. Perceived exertion in working capacity tests. In: Gunnar B, editor. Borg's perceived exertion and pain scales. 1st edition. Champaign (IL): Human Kinetics Publishers; 1998. p. 54–62.
79. Pollock ML, Franklin BA, Balady GJ, et al. Resistance exercise in individuals with and without cardiovascular disease: benefits, rationale, safety, and prescription: an advisory from the Committee on Exercise, Rehabilitation, and Prevention, Council on Clinical Cardiology, American Heart Association. Circulation 2000; 101:828–33.
80. King ML, Williams MA, Fletcher GF, et al. Medical director responsibilities for outpatient cardiac rehabilitation/secondary prevention programs: a scientific statement from the American Heart Association/American Association for Cardiovascular and Pulmonary Rehabilitation. Circulation 2005;112:3354–60.
81. Adams BJ, Carr JG, Ozonoff A, et al. Effect of exercise training in supervised cardiac rehabilitation programs on prognostic variables from the exercise tolerance test. Am J Cardiol 2008;101:1403–7.
82. Balady GJ, Jette D, Scheer J, et al. Changes in exercise capacity following cardiac rehabilitation in patients stratified according to age and gender: results of the Massachusetts Association of Cardiovascular and Pulmonary Rehabilitation Muticenter Database. J Cardiopulm Rehabil 1996;16(1):38–46.

83. Sakuragi S, Takagi S, Suzuki S, et al. Patients with large myocardial infarction gain a greater improvement in exercise capacity after exercise training than those with small to medium infarction. Clin Cardiol 2003;26(6):280–6.
84. Artham SM, Lavie CJ, Milani RV. Cardiac rehabilitation programs markedly improve high-risk profiles in coronary patients with high psychological distress. South Med J 2008;101:262–7.
85. Lavie CJ, Milani RV. Effects of cardiac rehabilitation programs on exercise capacity, coronary risk factors, behavioral characteristics, and quality of life in a large elderly cohort. Am J Cardiol 1995;76:177–9.
86. Hakim AA, Petrovith H, Burchfiel CM, et al. Effects of walking on mortality among nonsmoking retired men. N Engl J Med 1998;338:94–9.
87. Williams MA, Fleg JL, Ades PA, et al. Secondary prevention of coronary heart disease in the elderly (with emphasis on patients >=75 years of age): an American Heart Association Scientific Statement from the Council on Clinical Cardiology Subcommittee on exercise, cardiac rehabilitation, and prevention. Circulation 2002;105:1735–43.
88. Shanfield SB. Return to work after an acute myocardial infarction: a review. Heart Lung 1990;19:109–17.
89. Samkange-Zeeb F, Altenhöner T, Berg G, et al. Predicting non-return to work in patients attending cardiac rehabilitation. Int J Rehabil Res 2006;29:43–9.
90. Palatsi I. Feasibility of physical training after myocardial infarction and its effect on return to work, morbidity and mortality. Acta Med Scand Suppl 1976;599:7–84.
91. Hall HP, Wiseman VL, King MT, et al. Economic evaluation of a randomized trial of early return to normal activities versus cardiac rehabilitation after myocardial infarction. Heart Lung Circ 2002;11:10–8.
92. Schiller E, Baker J. Return to work after a myocardial infarction: Evaluation of planned rehabilitation and of a predictive rating scale. Med J Aust 1976;1:859–62.
93. Phillips L, Harrison T, Houck P. Return to work and the person with heart failure. Heart Lung 2004;34(2):79–88.
94. Simchen E, Naveh I, Zitser-Gurevich Y, et al. Is participation in cardiac rehabilitation programs associated with better quality of life and return to work after coronary artery bypass operations? Isr Med Assoc J 2001;3:399–403.
95. Mital A, Shrey D, Govindaraju M, et al. Accelerating the return to work chances of coronary heart disease patients: part 1—development and validation of a training programme. Disabil Rehabil 2000;11:604–20.
96. Brown AD, Garber AM. Cost effectiveness of coronary heart disease prevention strategies in adults. Pharmacoeconomics 1998;14(1):27–48.
97. Briffa TG, Eckermann SD, Griffiths AD. Cost-effectiveness of rehabilitation after an acute coronary event: a randomized controlled trial. Med J Aust 2005;183(9):450–5.
98. Levin L, Perk J, Hedback B. Cardiac rehabilitation—a cost analysis. J Intern Med 1991;230:427–34.
99. Oldridge N, Furlong W, Feeny D, et al. Economic evaluation of cardiac rehabilitation soon after acute myocardial infarction. Am J Cardiol 1993;72:154–61.
100. Ades PA, Pashkow FJ, Nestor JR. Cost-effectiveness of cardiac rehabilitation after myocardial infarction. J Cardiopulm Rehabil 1997;17:222–31.
101. Suaya JA, Shepard DS, Norman ST, et al. Use of cardiac rehabilitation by Medicare beneficiaries after myocardial infarction or coronary bypass surgery. Circulation 2007;116:1653–62.
102. Thomas RJ, Houston Miller N, Lamendola C, et al. National survey on gender differences in cardiac rehabilitation programs: patient characteristics and enrollment patterns. J Cardiopulm Rehabil 1996;16:402–12.

103. Harlan WR III, Sandler SA, Lee KL, et al. Importance of baseline functional and socioeconomic factors for participation in cardiac rehabilitation. Am J Cardiol 1995;76:36–41.
104. Bittner V, Sanderson B, Breland J, et al. Referral patterns to a university-based cardiac rehabilitation program. Am J Cardiol 1999;83:252–5.
105. Ades PA, Waldmann ML, Polk DM, et al. Referral patterns and exercise response in the rehabilitation of female coronary patients aged >=62 years. Am J Cardiol 1992;69:1422–5.
106. Ades PA, Waldmann ML, McCann WJ, et al. Predictors of cardiac rehabilitation participation in older coronary patients. Arch Intern Med 1992;152:1033–5.
107. Thomas RJ. Cardiac rehabilitation/secondary prevention programs: a raft for the rapids: why have we missed the boat? Circulation 2007;116:1644–6.
108. Carlson JJ, Johnson JA, Franklin BA, et al. Program participation, exercise adherence, cardiovascular outcomes, and program cost of traditional versus modified cardiac rehabilitation. Am J Cardiol 2000;86:17–23.
109. Oldridge N, Furlong W, Perkins A, et al. Community or patient preferences for cost-effectiveness of cardiac rehabilitation: does it matter? Eur J Cardiovasc Prev Rehabil 2008;15(5):608–15.
110. Taylor RS, Watt A, Dalal HM. Home-based cardiac rehabilitation versus hospital-based rehabilitation: a cost effectiveness analysis. Int J Cardiol 2007;119(2):196–201.
111. Jolly K, Taylor R, Lip GY, et al. The Birmingham Rehabilitation Uptake Maximisation study (BRUM): a randomised controlled trial comparing home-based with centre-based cardiac rehabilitation. Heart 2009;95(1):36–42.

Cardiovascular Disease in Persons with Spinal Cord Dysfunction—An Update on Select Topics

Jelena N. Svircev, MD[a,b,*]

KEYWORDS

- Spinal cord injuries • Cardiovascular diseases
- Dyslipidemias • Diabetes mellitus
- Peripheral vascular diseases • Amputation

As knowledge of spinal cord injury (SCI) and its consequences continue to increase, care delivered to individuals with SCI has improved significantly. This has translated to decreased mortality rates of persons with SCI over the preceding five decades.[1–3] However, the natural course of aging can bring an onset of new medical problems that differ from those that resulted at the time of immediate injury or illness. This includes the increased risk and complications resulting from cardiovascular disease (CVD), of which coronary heart disease (CHD) is a subset. The purposes of this article are to discuss the prevalence of CVD in persons with chronic SCI, to emphasize the scope of the problem, and to highlight particular areas of interest. A number of thorough reviews have been completed detailing each of the subject areas covered in this article. The reader is referred to these reviews to gain additional insight into the challenges of the issues discussed. The reader is further directed to a multitude of other sources addressing cardiovascular issues that predominantly occur in setting of acute and subacute SCI (eg, neurogenic shock, deep venous thrombosis).

EPIDEMIOLOGY

Historically, dysfunction of the renal and urinary tract systems were the leading causes of mortality in persons with SCI.[2,3] Improvements in the management of neurogenic

This work was supported by the Department of Veterans Affairs. The views expressed in this article are those of the author and do not necessarily reflect the position or policy of the Department of Veterans Affairs.

[a] Department of Rehabilitation Medicine, University of Washington, 1959 NE Pacific Street, Box 356490, Seattle, WA 98195, USA

[b] Department of Veterans Affairs, Spinal Cord Injury Service, Puget Sound Health Care System, 1660 S. Columbian Way—SCI 128, Seattle, WA 98108, USA

* Department of Veterans Affairs, Puget Sound Health Care System, Spinal Cord Injury Service, 1660 S. Columbian Way—SCI 128, Seattle, WA 98108, USA.

E-mail address: jsvircev@u.washington.edu

Phys Med Rehabil Clin N Am 20 (2009) 737–747
doi:10.1016/j.pmr.2009.06.012
1047-9651/09/$ – see front matter. Published by Elsevier Inc.

pmr.theclinics.com

bladder had led to a decrease in mortality from renal and urinary tract complications.[1–3] Although the precise prevalence is not known, it is believed that CVD accounts for a significant proportion of morbidity and mortality in individuals with SCI. Ischemic and nonischemic heart disease is second only to pneumonia and respiratory system diseases as the underlying cause of mortality in individuals with SCI.[1,3] DeVivo and Stover[1] reported that ischemic and nonischemic heart disease accounts for 18.7% of all deaths of known cause in individuals with SCI. In fact, heart disease is the second most common underlying cause of death in persons with tetraplegia, and the leading underlying cause of death in persons with paraplegia or Frankel D level of injury.[1] Combined, ischemic and nonischemic heart disease are the leading underlying causes of death in persons more than 5 years post injury.[1] Whiteneck and colleagues[2] reported that cardiovascular diseases were the most frequent causes of death among persons with SCI more than 30 years of age (46%) and more than 60 years of age (35%). This data is supported by a recent prospective study which suggested that diseases of the circulatory system were the most common (40%) underlying and contributing cause of death in individuals at least 1 year post injury.[4]

Heart disease is the leading cause of death in the United States.[5] The standardized mortality ratio (SMR) can be used to compare mortality rates for persons with SCI to that of the general population. DeVivo and Stover[1] reported no increased risk of mortality due to ischemic heart disease in individuals with SCI (SMR = 1.2), but a significant increase in mortality due to nonischemic heart disease (SMR = 6.4). Garshick and colleagues[4] demonstrated nonsignificant increases in SMR in disease of the heart (SMR = 0.59) or other diseases of the circulatory system (SMR = 1.49). However, both studies may be limited by availability of follow-up data or small numbers of deaths. A recent review of existing literature determined that there is no indication that individuals with SCI are at markedly greater risk for cardiovascular morbidity and mortality than able-bodied adults.[6] Although the prevalence of CVD in individuals with SCI may not be increased, its place as the leading cause of death suggests that the prevention of CVD in persons with SCI is as critical to the maintenance of health as it is in the able-bodied population. However, diagnosis and treatment of CVD in individuals with SCI present challenges not encountered in the noninjured people.

These studies provide valuable insight into the causes of death in persons with SCI. Current focus lies on the identification and prevention of CHD. Unfortunately, both identification and prevention of CVD in individuals with SCI is challenging. The ability of a person with SCI, particularly a higher-level injury, to report an ischemic event may be limited because of interrupted sensory pathways. Noninvasive cardiac stress testing has revealed that 63% to 65% of subjects have evidence of silent myocardial ischemia after dipyridamole administration and thallium-201 myocardial perfusion single-photon emission computed tomography imaging.[7–9] A cardiac event can pass unnoticed in some individuals.

CARDIOVASCULAR RECOMMENDATIONS IN THE GENERAL POPULATION

The Third Report of the Expert Panel on Detection, Evaluation, and Treatment of High Blood Cholesterol in Adults (ATP III) summarizes the current recommendations for management of elevated serum cholesterol levels in the general population.[10] The recommendations are based on levels of serum low-density lipoprotein (LDL) cholesterol and are influenced by the coexistence of CHD and the number of cardiac risk factors. CHD risk factors include diabetes mellitus, symptomatic carotid artery disease, peripheral artery disease, abdominal aortic aneurysm, cigarette smoking, hypertension, low-serum high-density lipoprotein (HDL) cholesterol levels, family history of premature CHD, and age ($\geq$45 years men, $\geq$55 years women). Risk estimates are established by determining a risk category for an individual, which serves as a basis for the treatment guidelines.

CARDIOVASCULAR CONCERNS IN SCI

Contributing to the increased risk for CVD in persons with SCI is the fact that nearly all cardiovascular risk factors are increased in individuals with SCI. Their patterns of dyslipidemia place them at risk for the development of arteriosclerosis. Increased rates of diabetes, impaired glucose tolerance, metabolic syndrome, and obesity contribute to the development of CVD, all conditions that are worsened by physical inactivity. The ability to modify cardiac risk factors, such as increasing activity level, may be difficult or extremely limited. Additionally, a number of consequences of SCI impart additional potential risk to these individuals, such as blood pressure abnormalities and cardiac rhythm disturbances.

LIPID METABOLISM

Abnormalities in lipid profiles play a significant role in the development of CHD. Depressed HDL cholesterol and elevated LDL cholesterol are risk factors for CHD.[10,11] Irregularities in lipid profiles are commonly seen in the setting of SCI.[6,12–18] Although consensus has not been reached on the impact of SCI on lipid profiles, agreement has been achieved on specific points. It is generally accepted that HDL cholesterol levels are depressed in individuals with SCI.[6,12–18] In one study, HDL cholesterol levels in persons with paraplegia or tetraplegia were lower compared with controls (37 $\pm$ 1 or 40 $\pm$ 1 versus 48 $\pm$ 2mg/dL).[12] Thirty-seven percent of subjects with SCI had HDL cholesterol levels less than 35mg/dL,[12] suggesting more stringent recommendations for target lipid levels.[10,11] Forty percent of individuals with SCI and LDL cholesterol levels between 130 and 160mg/dL also had serum HDL cholesterol levels below 35mg/dL.[12] In this subgroup, the HDL cholesterol level would have been undetected if lipoprotein profiles were only tested to record total cholesterol levels. Total serum cholesterol levels are often lower in persons with SCI, in part owing to depressed HDL cholesterol levels.[12,15] Neurologic level of injury appears to impact cholesterol levels in SCI.[13] Serum HDL cholesterol was lower in persons with tetraplegia versus paraplegia,[13,17] and the group with tetraplegia had a higher proportion of subjects with serum HDL cholesterol levels less than 35mg/dL than those with paraplegia.[13] A significant inverse relationship was found for the degree of neurologic deficit and mean serum HDL cholesterol levels; individuals with motor complete injury had lower levels of HDL than those with motor incomplete injuries within the subgroups of tetraplegia and paraplegia.[13] This suggests that greater severity of neurologic injury correlates with increased abnormalities in lipid profiles.

Ethnicity and gender are believed to have an effect on lipid profiles in persons with SCI.[14,15] In a study of 600 subjects with chronic SCI, the mean serum HDL cholesterol was found to be significantly higher in an African American group studied when compared with a white and Latino group.[14] White and Latino males with SCI, but not females or African American males, were found to have lower HDL cholesterol levels than able bodied sedentary control subjects.[15] Some studies suggest that mean serum LDL cholesterol levels are not significantly different in individuals with SCI when compared with controls,[12] while others report that LDL cholesterol, total cholesterol, and triglyceride levels are lower in individuals with SCI compared with control groups.[6,15] Increased activity level appears to have a favorable affect on lipid levels. De Groot and colleagues[19] noted that serum HDL cholesterol levels were significantly related to all measured physical capacity measures, including peak oxygen uptake, peak power output, and sum of handheld dynamometry measurements. This suggests that improving physical capacity by increasing physical activity in individuals with SCI may improve lipid profile, thereby reducing the risk of CHD. At the present time, literature suggests increased activity levels, in addition to smoking cessation and pharmacologic treatment may reduce CVD risk, although studies to clearly support this in the SCI population are needed.[20]

SMOKING AND SCI

Smoking is recognized as a risk factor for CHD in the general population. In addition to the well-accepted association of cigarette smoking with cancer and respiratory complications, smoking is believed to be associated with reduced HDL cholesterol, by mechanisms that are not clearly understood.[21,22] This may compound the already reduced levels of HDL cholesterol noted in individuals with SCI. Additionally, individuals with SCI may experience deterioration in pulmonary status as the result of smoking to a greater degree than the general population. This is supported by alterations in pulmonary function testing in smokers with SCI, such as reduced forced expiratory volume in 1 second and peak expiratory flow rate,[23] reduced ratio of forced expired volume in 1 second to forced vital capacity,[24] and increased functional residual capacity and residual volume.[25] Smoking may also be a risk factor for the development of pressure ulcers[26] and is associated with a higher incidence and more extensive pressure sores in individuals with SCI.[27] Further, smoking contributes to overall decreased self-reported health-related quality of life.[28]

DIABETES MELLITUS AND IMPAIRED GLUCOSE TOLERANCE

Diabetes mellitus is an independent risk factor for CVD[11] and reduction of CVD risk factors in persons with SCI and diabetes is critical. It is estimated that 13.4% to 22% of people with SCI have diabetes.[29–32] In a study of 100 veterans with SCI and 50 able-bodied control subjects, 22% of veterans with SCI were diabetic compared with 6% of control subjects.[29] Eighty two percent of able-bodied control subjects had normal glucose tolerance compared with 38% of individuals with tetraplegia and 50% of those with paraplegia.[29] Elevated levels of serum glucose and insulin are noted in response to oral glucose tolerance testing.[29,30,33,34] Bauman and Spungen[30] reported that after an oral glucose load in subjects with chronic SCI, 13.4% met criteria for the diagnosis of diabetes mellitus and 28.8% had impaired glucose tolerance. Of note, in this study, the diagnosis of diabetes would not have been made in 19 of 27 subjects based on fasting serum glucose values, suggesting that fasting serum glucose levels are inadequate for diagnosing diabetes in this population. Because the average fasting plasma glucose is only mildly elevated or within average range in people with SCI, it is believed that insulin resistance is the major factor responsible for glucose intolerance.[20] Data suggests that abnormalities in carbohydrate handling occurred at younger ages in those with SCI.[29] Veterans 50 to 64 years of age have twice the likelihood of having diabetes as those 50 years or younger. Veterans over 65 years of age are three times as likely to have diabetes as those under 50 years of age.[31] There is conflicting data relating to the neurologic level of injury and diabetes. In SCI veterans, it was found that those with paraplegia had a higher proportion of diabetes (17.2%) than those with tetraplegia (12.3%).[31] However, Bauman and colleagues,[30] found that more subjects with complete tetraplegia demonstrated a disorder of carbohydrate metabolism than other neurologic deficit subgroups. Ethnicity may play a role in the development of diabetes in individuals with SCI; Banerjea and colleagues[31] reported that blacks were 53% and Hispanics 74% more likely to have diabetes than were whites. Gender may also play a role in the development of diabetes and impaired glucose tolerance; it was noted that plasma insulin levels were higher in males than females at intermediate time points following an oral glucose load, suggesting a relative state of insulin resistance.[30] When diabetes occurs in persons with SCI, those with diabetes had twice the likelihood of macrovascular and microvascular complications than those without diabetes.[31]

A higher body fat content was found to be strongly associated with higher peak serum glucose and plasma insulin levels.[30,33] The loss of lean tissue mass has been demonstrated to occur in persons with SCI.[33,35,36] Additionally, the muscle tissue that remains has been demonstrated to contain a fourfold higher intramuscular fat percentage than in able bodied subjects by magnetic resonance imaging.[33] This loss of lean tissue mass may affect the way insulin is managed within the body and may further contribute to elevated glucose and insulin levels in individuals with SCI. The precise mechanism of insulin resistance is multifactorial and is in part due to denervated muscle, decreased lean muscle tissue, and increased fat tissue. There appears to be an association between glucose intolerance, insulin resistance, and SCI, related to inactivity and increased adiposity.[34] These adverse changes in body composition may negatively impact carbohydrate and lipid metabolism, which then increases the risk for CVD. Further studies are needed to evaluate the relative contributions of these specific factors to glucose intolerance, insulin resistance, and the development of diabetes. Diabetic care for individuals with SCI can improve with the implementation of coordinated, comprehensive care and increased health care provider awareness of the risks of CVD and diabetes this population. Rajan and colleagues[37] found that clinical outcomes, as measured in terms of glycosylated hemoglobin, blood pressure, and lipid values were improved in Veterans with SCI over a 3-year period for those receiving care at a Veterans Affairs Medical Center, either within the SCI system of care or primary care setting.

METABOLIC SYNDROME AND SCI

Metabolic syndrome has been defined by ATP III as a constellation of risk factors, including abdominal obesity, atherogenic dyslipidemia (elevated triglycerides, small LDL cholesterol particles, low HDL cholesterol), elevated blood pressure, insulin resistance (with or without glucose intolerance), and prothrombotic and proinflammatory states.[10] The ATP III recognizes this syndrome as a secondary target of risk-reduction therapy, after the primary target—LDL cholesterol.[10] Metabolic syndrome and insulin resistance was found to be present in 22.6% to 55% of people with SCI.[18,32] Unfortunately, criteria for the determination of metabolic syndrome in individuals with SCI have not been adequately defined, in part because of the limitations of addressing the unique characteristics of individuals with SCI with a definition that is suitable for the able-bodied population. For example, essential hypertension is not recognized as a widespread clinical problem in individuals with SCI, owing to blood pressure variability that exists with respect to the level of neurologic injury. Therefore, blood pressure measurements may have little diagnostic value in diagnosis metabolic syndrome in this population.[18] Additionally, healthy body mass index (BMI) values have been shown to underestimate adiposity in the SCI population.[38] These challenges limit the use of widely accepted definitions and emphasize the importance of a revised set of criteria that addresses the unique qualities of individuals with SCI.

OBESITY

Obesity is a significant challenge in individuals with SCI. Not only does it contribute to heightened risk of CVD, but it also plays a role in the development of pressure ulcers and can limit functional independence. BMI is determined by calculating the weight in kilograms divided by the square of the height in meters (kg/m2). The World Health Organization has defined "overweight" as a BMI equal to or more than 25, and "obesity" as a BMI equal to or more than 30.[39] Because body weight comprises lean tissue, fat tissue, and bone mass, in persons with varying proportions of these components obesity may not be accurately identified if BMI is used as a single measure.[39] Not only is there a potential for measurement error with the determination of weight and height in individuals with SCI, but evidence suggests that persons with SCI have greater fat mass and less lean tissue mass per unit BMI than age-matched, able-bodied control subjects.[35] Therefore, individuals with a high fat content may not appear obese, because of the loss of lean tissue replaced by extra fat. Using the World Health Organization's definition of "overweight" and "obese," it has been estimated that 33% of individuals with SCI are overweight according to their BMI and 20% are obese.[40] Individuals with SCI were found to have higher total body fat percentage and greater trunk fat when measured by dual radiograph (x-ray) absorptiometry (DEXA).[35] Adults with chronic SCI were found to have significantly more total adipose tissue and visceral adipose tissue than able-bodied adults matched for age, sex, and waist circumference by computed tomography scanning; this pattern of adipose distribution may place persons with SCI at particular risk for diabetes and CHD.[41] Abdominal visceral adipose tissue is characterized by very active lipolysis. High fatty acid levels reduce the uptake of insulin by hepatocytes, leading to increased insulin levels; therefore, increased abdominal visceral adipose tissue is believed to be closely associated with hyperinsulinemia. Abdominal circumference was negatively correlated with HDL cholesterol levels and positively correlated with triglyceride levels in men with spinal cord injury.[17] A number of studies have recommended that SCI-specific classifications of obesity be determined.[38,40,42] Some have proposed lowering the cutoffs for BMI for persons with SCI.[38,40] Weaver and colleagues[40] adjusted the BMI cutoffs and reported that the number of overweight and obese cases increased to 37 and 31 percent, respectively. Edwards and colleagues[41] demonstrated that waist circumference was highly correlated with visceral adipose tissue in persons with SCI. They advocated for the routine measurement of waist circumference at the lowest rib, rather than use of BMI, as a measure of abdominal obesity and a method of detecting CHD risk in this population. Estimates of percent body fat have been calculated using regression equations incorporating BMI values and DEXA measurements of body fat in persons with SCI,[30] but the validity of these equations has yet to be confirmed. Clearly, there is no consensus on a clinically useful measure of obesity for people with SCI and further investigation is needed.

SCI, PERIPHERAL VASCULAR DISEASE, AND LIMB LOSS

Limb loss can occur at the time of acute SCI, but is often seen as a consequence of secondary complications resulting from SCI, such as pressure sores, peripheral vascular disease, and lower limb fracture. One series estimated the overall amputation rate to be 1:10,000 SCI patients per year[43]; it is unclear if this value captured limb loss that occurred at time of SCI or in the setting of chronic SCI. Although pressure ulcers are the most common secondary complication in chronic SCI,[44] the incidence of limb loss in the SCI population due to pressure ulcers is unknown. The timely diagnosis of peripheral vascular disease (PVD) in persons with SCI is difficult owing to immobility and loss of sensation.[43,45] Individuals with unrecognized PVD often present with advanced limb ischemia leaving amputation as the best treatment option. Skin healing following surgical amputation is often challenging and prolonged because of unrecognized aortoiliac disease. Diagnosis of PVD is important, and a thorough vascular examination, including evaluation of femoral and pedal pulse should be part of the routine health maintenance evaluation in persons with SCI.

In the 1960s, some advocated for the amputation of "useless limbs," arguing that the procedure produced weight reduction and prevented development of pressure sores at the ankles and knees, and made transferring between wheelchair and bed easier. It was quickly recognized that complications from amputation were numerous and that indications for elective limb amputation should be the same for persons with SCI and in the able-bodied population.[46] Amputation of a limb is associated with increased mortality after SCI,[47] and the presence of limb loss should serve as an indicator for aggressive intervention in effort to reduce overall risk of mortality in these individuals. Limb salvage surgery for ischemic complications of the lower limbs in the setting of chronic SCI has been demonstrated to be successful in small case series,[48] but larger studies are needed to support routine surgical intervention for limb preservation in this population. Early revascularization procedures should be considered to avoid amputation or increase the success of skin healing postsurgery. Noninvasive vascular studies or angiograms should be considered if lower limb surgery is planned in persons with SCI.[45] Measurements of ankle-brachial index (ABI) may be a useful test for individuals with SCI in detecting PVD. A small, preliminary study compared individuals with chronic SCI and no risk factors or signs of PVD to an able-bodied control group and found no significant differences in ABI values.[49] Additional testing is required to confirm the findings and determine whether ABI correlates with the presence and severity of PVD in individuals with SCI.

Many factors need to be considered when the loss of limb in an individual with SCI is inevitable. An interdisciplinary team approach is best suited to address these issues. Leading the team is the person with SCI; if possible, he or she should be included in decision making during all phases of limb loss. Additional team members may include physiatrists, surgeons, prosthetists, orthotists, nurses, physical therapists (PT), occupational therapists (OT), recreational therapists, rehabilitation psychologists, dieticians, social workers, the individual's social support system, and practitioners from other medical disciplines.

The interdisciplinary team should consider functional consequences of limb loss in the setting of chronic SCI. The location of amputation along the length of the limb should be discussed. Longer residual lower limbs may improve pressure distribution while seated, but can place an individual at risk for complications associated with wound healing, contractures, and edema. A below-knee amputation may increase risk for skin breakdown at the distal limb if the individual has a knee flexion contracture. Ambulation potential and possible prosthetic options should be evaluated during the planning phase. The potential impact of lower limb loss on wheelchair seating should be considered, particularly in persons with a history of prior ischial, sacral, or trochanteric pressure ulcers.

The medical and nutritional status of the individual with SCI should be maximized to reduce postsurgical complications and support recovery and long-term health maintenance. The medical team can provide education to the individual with SCI and limb loss, and work with them to minimize risk factors that contribute to limb loss and CVD, such as poor diabetic control, uncontrolled hypertension, dyslipidemia, smoking, and obesity. Potential pain generators in a person with limb loss should be evaluated and the team should work to minimize pain. Treatment of pain may require consultation with PTs, OTs, surgeons, pharmacists, psychologists, prosthetists, orthotists, and anesthesiologists. Treatment options for pain may include education, behavioral interventions, medications, injections, surgery, therapeutic modalities, and complimentary or alternative therapies.

Nursing staff play a vital role increasing skin-protection measures and overall education with regard to maintaining skin integrity. During the postoperative period, they can work with the individual to implement protective positioning, such as avoiding maintained hip and knee flexion, elevating the residual limb for edema management, and reducing weight bearing through the residual limb. Nurses can provide and educate the individual with limb loss and SCI on compression wrapping of the residual limb, donning or doffing of a prosthesis, transfer techniques, and placement of urinary drainage bags. They can reinforce the importance of health problems associated with limb loss.

PTs, OTs, and recreational therapists play key roles in the management of limb loss and SCI. PTs and OTs assess and instruct in bed mobility and transfer training activities, and review wheelchair seating following lower limb loss. PTs can work with an individual with lower limb loss and SCI to assess gait potential with or without prosthesis, initiate gait training, and review mobility devices. PTs promote fitness and can provide exercise programs following limb loss for persons with SCI. OTs evaluate, provide, and train individuals in the use of adaptive equipment, including bathroom equipment, dressing aids, hygiene or skin protection tools, home modifications, and mobility devices. They can provide education and instruction on functional mobility and assistive devices for sexual activities. Recreational therapists can provide education and training in recreational activities and recreational equipment selection that will minimize complications with residual or intact limbs. They can teach a person with limb loss and SCI to identify potential aspects of recreational equipment and the environment that may affect skin integrity. They promote fitness activities and can instruct in how and where to access fitness programs. Recreational therapists can discuss the impact of limb loss and SCI on community access and social integration. All three disciplines can reinforce the importance of skin care and preventative care of the residual and remaining limbs.

Prosthetic limbs should be considered in ambulatory and nonambulatory individuals with SCI. For ambulatory individuals, daily activity level should be considered in the selection and design of the prosthesis. For nonambulatory persons with SCI, a cosmetic prosthesis to maintain positive body image may be of value. PT and prosthetists can provide and educate the individual with SCI and limb loss in casting and fitting of the prosthesis and train in the use of a prosthetic limb, for either mobility or cosmetic purposes.

The potential emotional affect of limb loss in an individual with acute or chronic SCI should not be underappreciated. Rehabilitation psychologists, psychiatrists, and social workers are skilled at addressing the psychosocial needs of individuals with limb loss and SCI. These disciplines can address concerns about body image with particular awareness of culture factors, such as ethnicity, race, gender, socioeconomic factors, or belief system. They can assess the potential impact of limb loss in family and caregiver dynamics, and discuss sexual issues addressing both physical aspects of SCI and limb loss and sexual identity. Psychologists or psychiatrists can provide an individual with strategies that address adjustment and coping following limb loss. This may include an evaluation of emotional adjustment and need for interventions, such as counseling sessions, medications, and education. They can encourage communication between the individual and family and friends, and can facilitate peer support. Social workers can educate and advocate on behalf of the individual within and outside of the medical community with regard to social services and community resources. They can assess caregiving needs and provide education about caregiving resources. Social workers can review the need for environmental modifications and facilitate hospital discharge planning.

SUMMARY

CVD is a leading cause of death in individuals with SCI and the able-bodied population.[1–5] The quality of evidence regarding prevalence of CVD and associated risks, and outcomes resulting from the disorders in the SCI population is weak. Additionally, the functional consequence of cardiovascular disorders has been an underexplored area of investigation. Current evidence does not support that adults with SCI are at significantly greater risk for cardiovascular morbidity or mortality.[6] It has been recommended that providers use the same thresholds to define or treat lipid and carbohydrate abnormalities in individuals with SCI as in able-bodied people.[6] Yet, it is recognized that, because of physiologic differences, people with SCI may be more challenged in meeting the recommended targets for cholesterol levels, diabetic control, and activity level. Further studies are needed to investigate the disorders, risks, and treatment options of CVD and associated disorders and practical guidelines should be established to facilitate the maintenance of heath for individuals with SCI.

REFERENCES

1. DeVivo MJ, Stover SJ. Long-term survival and causes of death. In: Stover SL, Delisa JA, Whiteneck GG, editors. Spinal cord injury: clinical outcomes from the model systems. Gaithersburg: Aspen Publishers; 1995. p. 289–316.
2. Whiteneck GG, Charlifue MA, Frankel HL, et al. Mortality, morbidity, and psychosocial outcomes of persons spinal cord injured more than 20 years ago. Paraplegia 1992;30:617–30.
3. Frankel HL, Coll JR, Charlifue SW, et al. Long-term survival in spinal cord injury: a fifty year investigation. Spinal Cord 1998;36:266–74.
4. Garshick E, Kelley A, Cohen SA, et al. A prospective assessment of mortality in chronic spinal cord injury. Spinal Cord 2005;43:408–16.
5. Kung HC, Hoyert DL, Xu J, et al. Deaths: final data for 2005. Natl Vital Stat Rep 2008;56(10):1–120.
6. Wilt TJ, Carlson FK, Goldish GD, et al. Carbohydrate and lipid disorders and relevant considerations in persons with spinal cord injury. Evidence Report/Technology Assessment No 163 (Prepared by the Minnesota Evidence-based Practice Center under Contract No 290-02-0009). AHRQ Publication No. 08-E005. Rockville (MD): Agency for Healthcare Research and Quality; 2008.
7. Bauman WA, Raza M, Chayes Z, et al. Tomographic thallium-201 myocardial perfusion imaging after intravenous dipyridamole in asymptomatic subjects with quadriplegia. Arch Phys Med Rehabil 1993;74:740–4.
8. Bauman WA, Raza M, Supngen AM, et al. Cardiac stress testing with thallium-201 imaging reveals silent ischemia in individuals with paraplegia. Arch Phys Med Rehabil 1994;75:946–50.
9. Lee CS, Lu YH, Lee ST, et al. Evaluating the prevalence of silent coronary artery disease in asymptomatic patients with spinal cord injury. Int Heart J 2006;47: 325–30.
10. Expert Panel on Detection. Evaluation, and treatment of high blood cholesterol in adults. Executive Summary of the Third Report of the National Cholesterol Education Program (NCEP) Expert Panel of Detection, Evaluation, and Treatment of

High Blood Cholesterol in Adults (Adult Treatment Panel III). JAMA 2001;285: 2486–97.

11. Pearson TA, Blair SN, Daniels SR, et al. AHA guidelines for primary prevention of cardiovascular disease and stroke: 2002 update: consensus panel guide to comprehensive risk reduction for adult patients without coronary or other atherosclerotic vascular diseases. Circulation 2002;106:388–91.

12. Bauman WA, Spungen AM, Zhong YG, et al. Depressed serum high density lipoprotein cholesterol levels in veterans with spinal cord injury. Paraplegia 1992;30: 697–703.

13. Bauman WA, Adkins RH, Spungen AM, et al. The effect of residual neurological deficit on serum lipoproteins in individuals with chronic spinal cord injury. Spinal Cord 1998;36:13–7.

14. Bauman WA, Adkins RH, Spungen AM, et al. Ethnicity effect on the serum lipid profile in persons with spinal cord injury. Arch Phys Med Rehabil 1998;79: 176–80.

15. Bauman WA, Adkins RH, Spungen AM, et al. Is immobilization associated with an abnormal lipoprotein profile? Observations from a diverse cohort. Spinal Cord 1999;37:485–93.

16. Ozgurtas T, Alaca R, Gulec M, et al. Do spinal cord injuries adversely affect serum lipoprotein profiles? Mil Med 2003;168:545–7.

17. Maki KC, Briones ER, Langbein WE, et al. Associations between serum lipids and indicators of adiposity in men with spinal cord injury. Paraplegia 1995;33:102–9.

18. Jones LM, Legge M, Goulding A. Factor analysis of the metabolic syndrome in spinal cord-injured men. Metabolism 2004;53(10):1372–7.

19. De Groot S, Dallmeijer AJ, Post MWM, et al. The longitudinal relationship between lipid profiles and physical capacity in persons with a recent spinal cord injury. Spinal Cord 2008;46:344–51.

20. Bauman WA, Spungen AM. Coronary heart disease in individuals with spinal cord injury: assessment of risk factors. Spinal Cord 2008;46:466–76.

21. Ellison RC, Zhang Y, Qureshi MM, et al. Lifestyle determinants of high-density lipoprotein cholesterol: the National Heart, Lung, and Blood Institute Family Heart Study. Am Heart J 2004;147:529–35.

22. Ashen MD, Blumenthal RS. Low HDL cholesterol levels. N Engl J Med 2005;353: 1252–60.

23. Almenoff PL, Spungen AM, Lesser M, et al. Pulmonary function survey in spinal cord injury: influences of smoking and level and completeness of injury. Lung 1995;173:297–306.

24. Linn WS, Spungen AM, Gong H, et al. Smoking and obstructive lung dysfunction in persons with chronic spinal cord injury. J Spinal Cord Med 2003;26: 28–35.

25. Stepp EL, Brown R, Tun CG, et al. Determinants of lung volumes in chronic spinal cord injury. Arch Phys Med Rehabil 2008;89:1499–506.

26. Gélis A, Dupeyron A, Legros P, et al. Pressure ulcer risk factors in persons with spinal cord injury part 2: the chronic stage. Spinal Cord 2009:1–11.

27. Lamid S, El Ghatit AZ. Smoking, spasticity and pressure scores in spinal cord injured patients. Am J Phys Med 1983;62:300–6.

28. Smith BM, LaVela SL, Weaver FM. Health-related quality of life for veterans with spinal cord injury. Spinal Cord 2008;46:507–12.

29. Bauman WA, Spungen AM. Disorders of carbohydrate and lipid metabolism in veterans with paraplegia or quadriplegia: a model of premature aging. Metabolism 1994;43(6):749–56.

30. Bauman WA, Adkins RH, Spungen AM, et al. The effect of residual neurological deficit on oral glucose tolerance in persons with chronic spinal cord injury. Spinal Cord 1999;37:765–71.
31. Banerjea R, Sambamoorthi U, Weaver F, et al. Risk of stroke, heart attack, and diabetes complications among veterans in spinal cord injury. Arch Phys Med Rehabil 2008;89:1448–53.
32. Lee MY, Myers J, Hayes A, et al. C-reactive protein, metabolic syndrome, and insulin resistance in individuals with spinal cord injury. J Spinal Cord Med 2005;28:20–5.
33. Elder CP, Apple DF, Bickel CS. Intramuscular fat and glucose tolerance after spinal cord injury—a cross-sectional study. Spinal Cord 2004;42:711–6.
34. Duckworth WC, Solomon SS, Jallepalli P, et al. Glucose intolerance due to insulin resistance in patients with spinal cord injuries. Diabetes 1980;29:906–10.
35. Jones LM, Goulding A, Gerrard DF. DEXA: a practical and accurate tool to demonstrate total and regional bone loss, lean tissue loss and fat mass gain in paraplegia. Spinal Cord 1998;36:637–40.
36. Spungen AM, Adkins RH, Stewart CA, et al. Factors influencing body composition in persons with spinal cord injury: a cross-sectional study. J Appl Physiol 2003;95:2398–407.
37. Rajan S, Hammond MC, Goldstein B. Trends in diabetes mellitus indicators in veterans with spinal cord injury. Am J Phys Med Rehabil 2008;87:468–77.
38. Jones LM, Legge M, Goulding A. Healthy body mass index values often underestimate body fat in men with spinal cord injury. Arch Phys Med Rehabil 2003; 84:1068–71.
39. Obesity: preventing and managing the global epidemic. Report of a WHO consultation. World Health Organ Tech Rep Ser 2000;894(i–xii):1–253.
40. Weaver FM, Collins EG, Kurichi J, et al. Prevalence of obesity and high blood pressure in veterans with spinal cord injuries and disorders. Am J Phys Med Rehabil 2007;86:22–9.
41. Edwards LA, Bugaresti JM, Buchholz AC. Visceral adipose tissue and the ratio of visceral to subcutaneous adipose tissue are greater in adults with than in those without spinal cord injury, despite matching waist circumferences. Am J Clin Nutr 2008;87(3):600–7.
42. Buchholz AC, Bugaresti JM. A review of body mass index and waist circumference as markers of obesity and coronary heart disease risk in persons with chronic spinal cord injury. Spinal Cord 2005;45:513–8.
43. Grundy DJ, Silver JR. Amputation for peripheral vascular disease in the paraplegia and tetraplegic. Paraplegia 1983;21:305–11.
44. McKinley WO, Jackson AB, Cardenas DD, et al. Long-term medical complications after traumatic spinal cord injury: regional model systems analysis. Arch Phys Med Rehabil 1999;80(11):1402–10.
45. Yokoo KM, Kronon M, Lewis VL Jr, et al. Peripheral vascular disease in spinal cord injury patients: a difficult diagnosis. Ann Plast Surg 1996;37:495–9.
46. Ohry A, Heim M, Steinbach TV, et al. The needs and unique problems facing spinal cord injured persons after limb amputation. Paraplegia 1983;21:260–3.
47. Krause JS, Carter RE, Pickelsimer EE, et al. A prospective study of health and risk of mortality after spinal cord injury. Arch Phys Med Rehabil 2008;89:1482–91.
48. Dalman RL, Harris EJ, Walker MT, et al. Limb salvage surgery in spinal cord injury. Ann Vasc Surg 1998;12:60–4.
49. Grew M, Kirshblum SC, Wood K, et al. The ankle brachial index in chronic spinal cord injury: a pilot study. J Spinal Cord Med 2000;23(4):284–8.

Index

Note: Page numbers of article titles are in **boldface** type.

Phys Med Rehabil Clin N Am 20 (2009) 749–757
doi:10.1016/S1047-9651(09)00073-4
1047-9651/09/$ – see front matter © 2009 Elsevier Inc. All rights reserved.

pmr.theclinics.com

Moving?

Make sure your subscription moves with you!

To notify us of your new address, find your **Clinics Account Number** (located on your mailing label above your name), and contact customer service at:

Email: journalscustomerservice-usa@elsevier.com

800-654-2452 (subscribers in the U.S. & Canada)
314-447-8871 (subscribers outside of the U.S. & Canada)

Fax number: 314-447-8029

Elsevier Health Sciences Division
Subscription Customer Service
3251 Riverport Lane
Maryland Heights, MO 63043

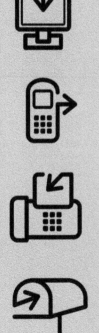

*To ensure uninterrupted delivery of your subscription, please notify us at least 4 weeks in advance of move.

United States Postal Service

Statement of Ownership, Management, and Circulation
(All Periodicals Publications Except Requestor Publications)

1. Publication Title	2. Publication Number	3. Filing Date
Physical Medicine and Rehabilitation Clinics of North America	0 0 9 9 - 2 4 3	9/15/09

4. Issue Frequency	5. Number of Issues Published Annually	6. Annual Subscription Price
Feb, May, Aug, Nov	4	$213.00

7. Complete Mailing Address of Known Office of Publication (Not printer) (Street, city, county, state, and ZIP+4®)

Elsevier Inc.
360 Park Avenue South
New York, NY 10010-1710

Contact Person
Stephen Bushing

Telephone (Include area code)
215-239-3688

8. Complete Mailing Address of Headquarters or General Business Office of Publisher (Not printer)

Elsevier Inc., 360 Park Avenue South, New York, NY 10010-1710

9. Full Names and Complete Mailing Addresses of Publisher, Editor, and Managing Editor (Do not leave blank)

Publisher (Name and complete mailing address)

John Schrefer, Elsevier, Inc., 1600 John F. Kennedy Blvd. Suite 1800, Philadelphia, PA 19103-2899

Editor (Name and complete mailing address)

Catherine Bewick, Elsevier, Inc., 1600 John F. Kennedy Blvd. Suite 1800, Philadelphia, PA 19103-2899

Managing Editor (Name and complete mailing address)

Deb Dellapena, Elsevier, Inc., 1600 John F. Kennedy Blvd. Suite 1800, Philadelphia, PA 19103-2899

10. Owner (Do not leave blank. If the publication is owned by a corporation, give the name and address of the corporation immediately followed by the names and addresses of all stockholders owning or holding 1 percent or more of the total amount of stock. If not owned by a corporation, give the names and addresses of the individual owners. If owned by a partnership or other unincorporated firm, give its name and address as well as those of each individual owner. If the publication is published by a nonprofit organization, give its name and address.)

Full Name	Complete Mailing Address
Wholly owned subsidiary of	4520 East-West Highway
Reed/Elsevier, US holdings	Bethesda, MD 20814

11. Known Bondholders, Mortgagees, and Other Security Holders Owning or Holding 1 Percent or More of Total Amount of Bonds, Mortgages, or Other Securities. If none, check box ☐ None

Full Name	Complete Mailing Address
N/A	

12. Tax Status (For completion by nonprofit organizations authorized to mail at nonprofit rates) (Check one)
The purpose, function, and nonprofit status of this organization and the exempt status for federal income tax purposes:
☐ Has Not Changed During Preceding 12 Months
☐ Has Changed During Preceding 12 Months (Publisher must submit explanation of change with this statement)

PS Form 3526, September 2007 (Page 1 of 3 (Instructions Page 3)) PSN 7530-01-000-9931 PRIVACY NOTICE: See our Privacy policy in www.usps.com

---

13. Publication Title	14. Issue Date for Circulation Data Below
Physical Medicine and Rehabilitation Clinics of North America	May 2009

15. Extent and Nature of Circulation		Average No. Copies Each Issue During Preceding 12 Months	No. Copies of Single Issue Published Nearest to Filing Date
a. Total Number of Copies (Net press run)		1788	1550
b. Paid Circulation (By Mail and Outside the Mail)	(1) Mailed Outside-County Paid Subscriptions Stated on PS Form 3541. (Include paid distribution above nominal rate, advertiser's proof copies, and exchange copies)	847	761
	(2) Mailed In-County Paid Subscriptions Stated on PS Form 3541 (Include paid distribution above nominal rate, advertiser's proof copies, and exchange copies)		
	(3) Paid Distribution Outside the Mails Including Sales Through Dealers and Carriers, Street Vendors, Counter Sales, and Other Paid Distribution Outside USPS®	276	258
	(4) Paid Distribution by Other Classes Mailed Through the USPS (e.g. First-Class Mail®)		
c. Total Paid Distribution (Sum of 15b (1), (2), (3), and (4))		1123	1019
d. Free or Nominal Rate Distribution (By Mail and Outside the Mail)	(1) Free or Nominal Rate Outside-County Copies Included on PS Form 3541	77	79
	(2) Free or Nominal Rate In-County Copies Included on PS Form 3541		
	(3) Free or Nominal Rate Copies Mailed at Other Classes Through the USPS (e.g. First-Class Mail)		
	(4) Free or Nominal Rate Distribution Outside the Mail (Carriers or other means)		
e. Total Free or Nominal Rate Distribution (Sum of 15d (1), (2), (3) and (4))		77	79
f. Total Distribution (Sum of 15c and 15e)		1200	1098
g. Copies not Distributed (See instructions to publishers #4 (page #3))		588	452
h. Total (Sum of 15f and g)		1788	1550
i. Percent Paid (15c divided by 15f times 100)		93.58%	92.81%

16. Publication of Statement of Ownership
If the publication is a general publication, publication of this statement is required. Will be printed ☐ Publication not required
in the November 2009 issue of this publication.

17. Signature and Title of Editor, Publisher, Business Manager, or Owner	Date
[signature] Joseph Patrick, Executive Director of Subscription Services	September 15, 2009

I certify that all information furnished on this form is true and complete. I understand that anyone who furnishes false or misleading information on this form or who omits material or information requested on the form may be subject to criminal sanctions (including fines and imprisonment) and/or civil sanctions (including civil penalties).

PS Form 3526, September 2007 (Page 2 of 3)

Printed and bound by CPI Group (UK) Ltd, Croydon, CR0 4YY

03/10/2024

01040462-0014